Heloise's
BEAUTY
B·O·O·K

Manufactured in the United States of America

Design by Rueith Ottiger/Levavi & Levavi

10 9 8 7 6 5 4 3 2

This book is printed on acid free paper. The paper in this book meets the guidelines for permanence and durability of the Committee on Production Guidelines for Book Longevity of the Council on Library Resources.

Library of Congress Cataloging in Publication Data

Heloise.
  Heloise's Beauty book.

  Bibliography: p. 321
  1. Beauty, Personal. 2. Clothing and dress. 3. Skin—Care and hygiene. 4. Reducing diets. 5. Exercise.
I. Title. II. Title: Beauty book.
RA778.H453 1985   646.7'042   84-24452
ISBN 0-87795-654-5 (alk. paper)

Dedicated to all women who want to look and feel their best and to my special husband, David, who makes it worth the effort when I do

CONTENTS

ACKNOWLEDGMENTS

Hugs and thanks to my dear friend and editor Judith Riven, who told me I could do this book.

To Marcy Meffert, editorial research assistant, guinea pig, and all around helper, for helping to put all of this information together.

To Joan O'Sullivan, senior editor at King Features, and Eleanor Johnson, senior editor at Arbor House, who made sure I crossed my *t*'s and dotted my *i*'s. So did I?

INTRODUCTION: A WORD FROM HELOISE

Since I was a tot, I've heard that "beauty is as beauty does." Maybe so, but strictly speaking, I think "beauty is as beauty does to herself." Very few of us can count on natural beauty to see us through; most of us need some retouching. Some of the world's greatest beauties have imperfect features—a large nose, small eyes, thin lips, and the like—or figures that don't measure up to beauty-contest standards. Why aren't we aware of such drawbacks? Because they've learned how to minimize imperfect features with makeup and to dress cleverly so their figures look fabulous.

Happily, this fine art of camouflage is not reserved for the rich and famous. Every woman can learn to retouch her personal portrait. That's what this book is all about. In it, I'm sharing how-to hints that will help you realize your full beauty potential. I've learned them from celebrated professionals and from readers of my Heloise column, and some are strictly personal tricks I've mastered via trial and error.

Whatever the hint, one thing is for sure: when it comes from your friend Heloise you can be certain you won't have to sell your car or take a second mortgage on your home to finance it. If there's one thing I believe, it's in getting things done as inexpensively, quickly, and easily as I can.

For example, in this book you will find recipes for "kitchen cosmetics" made with such things as mayonnaise, avocado, and/or olive oil, together or separately, not for a new chip dip, but to condition your hair. You'll find essential health hints, some that are absolutely free—like drinking six to eight glasses of water daily to moisturize your skin from within, to help your body flush away wastes, and to take the edge off your appetite when you diet. You'll learn all kinds of things, including the fact that all the "leather-necks" aren't in the U.S. Marine Corps; many can be found on the golf course, in gardens, and at poolside, basking in the sun and leatherizing more than just their necks, oblivious to the fact that the sun is their skin's worst enemy.

You'll also find hints on getting the most mileage from your wardrobe. The first step is to organize your closet so you can get dressed with the most style and the least trauma. Next you'll find specific advice on how to update, add to, and shop for a wardrobe that may be minimal but is planned to serve maximum needs.

Once you find the beauty routines that work best for you, the health-diet-exercise programs that make you feel great, the wardrobe that insures you look your best every day, you'll have in hand the real secret of beauty: a confident and positive attitude.

Believing that you're special puts a sparkle in your eyes and a spring in your step that even the best makeup job, face-lift surgery or vitamin tonic can't provide. So read on. Soon you'll be showing the world the most beautiful you—a new you.

Hugs,
Heloise

Chapter 1

STRICTLY PERSONAL

Don't worry, I'm not going literary on you, but whenever I think about skin, I think of what Mark Twain reportedly said one summer day: "It's so hot, I want to take off my skin and sit around in my bones." Well, sometimes I couldn't agree more. There are days when my skin looks dry, oily, broken out, or sunburned, and I feel as if I'd like to take it off, send it to the cleaners or some miracle worker, because I'd rather just sit around in my bones and not be seen at all.

But of course you and I can't do that. All we can do is slough off dead skin and try to take care of what we have. Believe me, if you take care of the skin you have, it will not only look good, but it will take care of itself. And you know what? It's the only skin you've got, so you'd better start now. One of my personal beauty habits gives my editor gray hairs at the very mention of it, but I'm going to tell you about it anyway.

I like to leave my mascara on for five or six days. You heard me right. I know a lot of women take their mascara off every night, and if you have any eye problems or allergies you *should*. I don't take mine off because I like the way my lashes look with a buildup of mascara on them. I use waterproof mascara, which barely smudges. People are always complimenting me on my lashes and asking me if they're real, so I must be doing something right!

While we're on the subject of personal beauty habits, here's another. But first let me say that, though it works for me, it's not likely to work for someone who doesn't have a steady hand. When I put on the first layer of mascara, I let it dry for thirty seconds or so before applying the next coat. Then, at thirty-second intervals, I apply several more coats. Here is the trick that turns my husband into a bundle of raw nerves. (He won't even come near the bathroom when I'm doing this.) Very, very carefully, I separate my lashes with a hatpin. Yes, a hatpin. This way, they don't get clumped together.

Where did I learn this beauty habit? My mother. She told me, "Well, this is what I do, but you really shouldn't do this because you might hurt yourself." And that's my advice to you, too. *Don't try it unless you have a very steady hand.*

Not *all* my beauty routines scare people. Most of the time, they are quite ordinary and probably not unlike some of your own. One thing we can all be grateful for is that we don't use the heavy cake makeup women wore years ago. With all that gunk on their faces, they had to use cold cream just to get it off. Today's lighter face makeup or foundation doesn't take much effort at all to remove.

Here's my basic routine: I wash my face well at night with a washcloth and a mild soap or heavy-fatted face soap. If I'm in a hotel, I use whatever is there—unless it's a deodorant soap. They're too drying for my face. After washing my face, I pat it dry and then put on a moisturizer. In the morning, I don't rub and scrub. I just splash my face with cold water and gently "wash" with a washcloth and water only. I don't need to use soap because my face is already clean. Afterward, I apply moisturizer and makeup.

Here's my two-minute makeup routine for those days I don't have time to "do it all the way." Since my office is my home, sometimes I don't get fully dressed to go to the office. If I'm working on a deadline, I may still be in my bathrobe or cutoffs and a T-shirt at one in the afternoon, but I always manage at least to take a swipe at my face.

First, I always keep an old makeup bottle filled with half makeup and half moisturizer; a few dots never fail to kill two birds with one stroke—and a few pats.

Then comes a touch of cream rouge or blusher on the cheeks. If you're out of blusher, you can put a dab of lipstick in your hand, add a drop of moisturizer, mix well, then pat it on your cheeks and blend. (It looks more natural than powder.)

If I have a blemish, or circles under my eyes, a quick touch with a cover-up usually does the trick.

The next step is the eyes. For fast work, I draw a line or two in the crease with a brown cream pencil, then smear or blend with the brush I use for brown powder eye shadow.

Then I use my old faithful toothbrush (ten years old) to comb through and separate my eyelashes before one or two quick run-throughs with mascara.

The final touches are a spritz of cologne and a dab of lip gloss. Then I brush my hair and I'm out the door.

I bet it's taken you longer to read this than it would to do it, so why don't you give it a try? A minute or two is well worth the effort. It makes me feel like I can face the world (and the world can face me).

My cleaning routine at the end of the day is pretty simple. First, I wash with soap and water and a cloth, because the slight roughness of the washcloth helps slough off those dead cells. If you don't slough off dead skin cells, you get a buildup that makes your makeup look terrible. You know the buildup I mean; the kind you have when you're about to peel from a sunburn. If you look closely at your skin with a magnifying mirror (don't panic!) you can sometimes actually see the dead skin that needs to be removed. Some cosmetologists say that getting rid of dead skin also helps make wrinkles and enlarged pores less noticeable. It makes sense to me.

When my face gets that "yucky" look from dead skin cell buildup, I try a five-minute facial, using the lotion made for removal of dead skin from feet and elbows. You rub it on and the dead skin just rolls off.

I find that this lotion is much better than regular use of cleansing grains and abrasive puffs. Why? Because I think using the harsher methods incorrectly or too often can be bad for your skin. I asked my dermatologist if it was safe to use the foot-and-elbow lotion on my face, and he said it's fine; but he did caution me that, as with all treatments for your face, it's important to avoid the eye area, because of its thinness and sensitivity. Be sure to test-spot it first.

But just because it's not for me, doesn't mean it's not for you. One of my research assistants thinks abrasive puffs are the greatest invention since the cotton swab. She's allergic to most ingredients used for facials and peels, and until she began to use abrasive puffs, she was constantly fighting clogged pores. This is a woman who is pushing fifty so hard she's about to knock it over, and she has to use a puff *gently* twice a day with medicated or "pure" soaps, especially on the oily sections of her skin, or the oil blocks pores and she gets blemishes. She says that these puffs wear out fast and can get very rough after about two months of use, so they should be discarded or transferred to the kitchen, where they can be used to scrub ceramic cookware—with baking soda, of course.

When I'm on the road for lectures or book-promotion tours and need to scrub my face, especially after wearing TV makeup day after day, I can't and don't carry along everything I use at home for beauty routines. What I do is sprinkle a lot of salt or sugar in my hand, and a little water, and then gently scrub my face. You can soap your face before using this gentle scrub, but always follow up by carefully rinsing (at least ten to fifteen splashes of water), followed with a slathering of moisturizer.

If you have an outbreak of blemishes or sores, skip your sloughing-off routine until it clears up. When you are paying special attention to your skin, don't forget shoulders and arms, especially if you are going to be wearing a strapless or revealing gown. Have you ever noticed how many women seem to have forgotten that their elbows need extra care? Well, maybe *you* don't have to look at your elbows, but *others* do. If you don't believe me, the next time you're at the beach or pool, check out other people's elbows and heels. Not a pretty picture, is it?

It doesn't matter how much money you pay for your clothes, how well you put yourself together, or how great your figure is, if you're walking around with scaly, gray, cracked "elephant" skin on your elbows, your whole appearance is spoiled. So take a moment to look at yourself in the mirror—from the rear—with your arms hanging straight down. That's how you look to others.

It's so easy to bleach and soften those elbows. Any time you squeeze lemons, save the little cups of lemon halves and spend about fifteen minutes resting your elbows in them while you read or think pleasant thoughts. Remember, maintenance is the key with all parts of your body—be sure to put extra lotion on *any* part of your body, including your elbows, that takes a little extra abuse and tends to get dry.

• *TESTING NEW PRODUCTS AND INGREDIENTS* •

I've already mentioned test spotting, but I'd like to take a moment to remind you that whenever you decide to try a new beauty product, whether it's from the store or your kitchen or your garden, it's a good idea to test it on a patch of skin. Think of it as a sort of "Captain, may I?" before you take that "giant step" of a whole treatment. This is especially important if you've had allergies or are sensitive to certain herbs or chemicals. Dermatologists recommend that people with allergies or sensitivities read labels carefully and select products containing the fewest ingredients—the idea being that the fewer the ingredients, the less the chances are that you'll get zapped by one that is incompatible with your body. One popular and inexpensive hand lotion lists as its active ingredients only glycerin, white petrolatum, and zinc oxide.

Don't underestimate the potency of beauty products. I used to have a problem with puffy eyes in the morning. It didn't seem to matter how much sleep I'd had, or what I'd eaten or drunk the night before. Then I heard that using too much eye cream or moisturizer around the eye area could cause puffiness. Well, I had my doubts, but I thought I'd try a little experiment anyway. I applied my moisturizer as usual, but only around one eye. Boy, oh boy, that was it! I had been putting too much eye cream around my eyes, and that's why they were so puffy in the morning. (I'll tell you more about puffy eyes in Chapter 4, "Rx for Eyes.")

You can experiment with new products, too. Here is a simple patch test that you can do at home before you try new makeup, soaps, herbal kitchen cosmetics, or especially hair dyes and bleaches, which seem to be a problem for a lot of people. (This test is excerpted from a book by Dr. Edward R. Pinckney, M.D. and Cathey Pinckney, *Do-It-Yourself Medical Testing: More than 100 Tests You Can Do at Home,* Facts on File, 1983.)

Apply a small dot of the product or herb—one no larger than a match head—to a half-inch square or circle of unmedicated gauze adhesive bandage. If the material is not liquid, mix it with one or two drops of water or mineral oil—the oil won't evaporate, so it may be better to use. Place the patch on a hair-free area of skin, such as the inside of your arm or elbow, or your back. Leave it there for forty-eight hours. Don't get it wet.

If the test area burns, itches, aches, or feels even a little bit irritated, remove the patch immediately and flush the area with water. If the irritation continues, get a nonprescription cortisone ointment from your pharmacist or see your doctor.

When you remove the patch, you should be able to gauge your degree of sensitivity (if any) to the material by the amount of redness, swelling, pimples, blisters, or itching that developed under the patch. If you are sensitive, you'll have a reaction within two to forty-eight hours after putting the patch in place; if you have no reaction, then it should be safe for you.

Allergies to drugs or foods seem to show up faster with this test than allergies to plants or pets.

If you are using this patch test for the first time, to get accurate results you'll have to use "control" patches. Don't panic—this may sound mighty scientific, but it really isn't. What it means is you want to make sure you aren't reacting to the bandage or something in your water or the mineral oil. So, in addition to the test patch, place two other patches on other skin locations—one dry, and one soaked in water or mineral oil, whichever you used for the test. Just make sure your control patches don't contain any of the material being tested.

Now this may seem like a lot of trouble, but think of the pain and misery if you took a bath in something that irritated your whole body! Or had to comb your hair after your scalp had blistered from a bleach or dye! It gives me goose bumps just to think about it! Any of you who have ever had such a reaction know how important testing is. A friend's scalp blistered after she tried a certain hair bleach, and she still gets the shivers and shakes when she walks past drugstore hair-coloring displays.

Chapter 2

YOUR SKIN: FACING UP TO BEAUTY

· SOAPS ·

You can't talk about skin without talking about soap. No matter what the lady behind the cosmetic counter says—many cosmetologists will lead you to believe that using soap on your face is only a little better than using paint stripper—washing with soap and water is still the most popular, effective way to clean your skin.

Finding the right soap for your skin is really a matter of trial and error. But as with all substances that you apply to your skin, the more ingredients they contain, the greater the likelihood of one being an irritant. Additives such as deodorants and perfumes seem to bother a lot of people. The climate affects skin, too, so you may find that you need different soaps at different times of the year. For example, in the summer your skin tends to absorb more dirt because you perspire more, and it is oilier. Cold weather dries out even the oiliest skin, so you will probably need moisturizers in the winter.

How can you match skin type and soap? It's simple. If you have dry skin, use a superfatted soap. Some glycerin soaps are good with dry skin, but not the ones containing alcohol, which is a drying ingredient. If you have dry skin you should probably wash only once daily in the winter (at night) and twice a day in the summer.

If you have oily skin, use any regular or deodorant soap. Avoid all soaps with oils or emollients. Acne soaps help certain types of blemished skins, but some may overdry skin that's only slightly oily, so if you have a real acne problem, ask your doctor to suggest the right soap for your skin. People with oily skin should wash twice a day in the winter and three times a day or more in the summer. Detergent soaps are generally good for oily skin. Contrary to what you've probably heard, detergent doesn't automatically mean it belongs in the kitchen or laundry. Some detergent soaps are actually milder than toilet soaps, and they certainly rinse off more easily. How can you tell if a soap is a detergent soap? If it lists sulfate or sulfonate among its ingredients.

Whatever your skin type, there is a *right* way to wash your face: wet it; lather up once, using only warm, not extremely hot or cold water; then rinse away every trace of soap with a soft washcloth. (Make sure it's clean!)

When you set out to buy soap, judging the quality can be a real adventure, because the packages and labels are often distracting and misleading. One magazine article claims that 10 percent of the soap's price is for the packaging, 20 percent for the fragrance, and 70 percent for the other ingredients.

Here are a few of the "families" of soaps you'll find in stores:

• *Fragrance Soaps:* those with herbs, flowers, spices, essences of perfumes
• *Pumice Soaps:* those with about 25 percent crushed volcanic rock, used to get out grit and grease
• *Skin-sensitive Soaps:* those containing special skin aids or those that eliminate known irritants from their formulas
• *Pure Soap:* it's up to you to figure out just what this means, but in general remember that calling a soap "pure" has come to mean only that it can be "pure" anything.

Some soaps have no colors or fragrances, and their scent comes from their basic ingredients.

Glycerin soaps are not all the same, because different glycerins are made to work in different water temperatures. Detergents, al-kalis, and acids may bother sensitive skins, and I've read that the more chemicals are added, the cheaper is the process for making the soap. If that's so, then really pure soap could justify a higher price tag.

Here are some definitions of soap terms that should help you read labels:

• *True Soap:* when a fat or oil is broken down into fatty acid and glycerin, the glycerin is removed (except in transparent soaps), and the fatty acid is neutralized with a caustic soda. The result is "true" soap. Ingredients such as oils, scents, coloring, and antibacterial agents can be added to this basic soap. Ivory soap, advertised as "99 and 44/100ths percent pure" is a good example of a pure soap.

• *Synthetic Soaps:* synthetic soaps are made from detergents, which come from petroleum materials, fatty acids, and other sources. They are less alkaline, work better in hard water, and don't leave a bathtub ring. They are found in bar, gel, and liquid forms and contain various additional ingredients for special purposes. As with "true" soaps, their effect upon your skin depends largely on the specific ingredients.

• *Milled Soaps* (you'll see the phrase "triple milled" on labels): about half of the toilet soaps, including synthetics, are milled, which means that soap chips are blended and compacted into bars. The color, texture, and distribution of added ingredients are consistent, and moisture is removed so that the bars will last longer.

• *Superfatted Soaps:* these soaps contain extra fats or oils, such as fatty acids, coconut oil, mineral oil, lanolin, and cocoa butter.

• *Transparent Soaps:* both scented and nonscented, these soaps contain 10 percent more glycerin, a humectant that is said to help your skin hold moisture. Some contain alcohol and will therefore dry out skin.

• *Deodorant Soaps:* these soaps contain additional fragrance to mask body odor, or antibacterial agents to inhibit odor-causing bacteria growth. Many deodorant soaps used to contain tribromo-salicylanilide (TBS), but this substance was found to cause sun sensitivity and has since been banned by the FDA.

• *Acne Soaps:* these soaps are *only* for people with very oily or blemish-prone skin. Why? They contain such ingredients as sulfur, salicylic acid, resorcinol, or benzoyl peroxide, which make them extremely drying. If you are sensitive to sulfur *read labels carefully*.

• *Liquid Soaps:* these are a combination of real and synthetic soaps, containing glycerin. Actually, in terms of their cleaning properties, liquid soaps are no different from other soaps. Most are synthetics and are popular because they help avoid the mess of slippery, dissolving bars.

• *Nonscented Soaps:* generally fragrance-free, these are best suited to people with sensitive skin or allergies.

• *Specialty Soaps:* these possess the same cleansing properties of other soaps, but look and smell different because they contain ingredients such as vegetable or fruit juices, vitamins, minerals, wheat germ, exotic perfumes, or oatmeal.

Most dermatologists agree that the best soaps are the simplest ones. Beware of soaps that claim to moisturize, protect, or lubricate your skin while cleaning it—they aren't on your face long enough to do all that. And expensive ingredients such as vitamin E or wheat germ oil are washed right down the drain with the suds. In general, sensitive skins may do better with baby soaps. When you're reading a soap's ingredients, remember that even the *relatives* of allergens may bother your skin.

The lesson here? Learn about your skin's needs. Choose your soap carefully and sensibly, and don't let fancy names and labels fool you.

• *CLEANSING CREAMS* •

You may find that the very same makeup demonstrator who acts as if soap and paint remover are poured from the same evil vat will sing the praises of cleansing cream. Cleansing creams are an updated version of the cold creams that women used to use to take off heavy cake makeup. Although cleansers possess many of the same chemical properties as soap, they do seem to do a better job of removing makeup. But most dermatologists contend that you don't need cleansers unless you wear heavy makeup and powder, or have dry skin that is irritated by soaps. Cleansing creams stick to your skin, are difficult to remove, and can clog your pores.

How do advertisers justify the use of cleansing creams? The sales pitch tells you that you need a variety of potions and lotions to clarify, tone, balance, and so forth. Actually, these products are astringents—solutions with alcohol or witch hazel—which make your skin feel tingly or give it a blush and which cause water to evaporate from your skin. Your skin will look smoother after application of an alcohol-based astringent, because alcohol makes your skin swell slightly; then pores shrink temporarily. Many dermatologists agree that even if you have very oily skin, you don't need astringents. You just need to wash your face more often.

• *WRINKLES* •

Now, you probably don't want to hear this, but I've researched this hateful topic thoroughly and I'm sorry to report that the only real "wrinkle remover" is an expert plastic surgeon. You can put things on your face that will make your skin temporarily swell up or tighten up, so that wrinkles don't show. You can put petrolatum (petroleum jelly) products on your wrinkles so that the shiny surface looks less wrinkled (that's how most wrinkle removers work); you can work on a positive, happy outlook so that the sparkle in your eyes detracts from your wrinkles. But only surgery will take the wrinkles away. Sorry, if that's not what you wanted to hear. I don't like it much either.

As for preventing wrinkles, there are two ways: you can avoid using your face expressively, so creases don't develop—not practical, and I'm not so sure your face wouldn't begin to droop anyway, after the muscles atrophy from disuse. It's fun to develop smile lines, and if there is any such thing as *good* lines, they're it.

The second way is more practical, but I'm sure some of you aren't going to like it either: stay out of the sun, or wear a sunscreen or full sunblock every time you are exposed to sunshine.

There. Not much fun is it? But the fact is that the sun speeds along the natural aging process of the skin. Wrinkles result from the deterioration of elastin and collagen, the tissues that make up the dermis (underlayer of skin) and keep skin supple and flexible. When these tissues deteriorate, the dermis gets loose, folds up under the epidermis (outer layer of skin), and then you have wrinkles, usually in the lines around your eyes or mouth—whatever you use the most for smiling, frowning—or, if you are a smoker, around your lips, where you pucker up to inhale. I know this is a mouthful, but if you understand the "whys" of wrinkles, maybe it would be easier to prevent them.

The FDA forbids mislabling of products, so cosmetic companies have dreamed up cutesy names for their wrinkle products, especially since they can't honestly use the term "wrinkle remover."

Wrinkle creams can make wrinkles diminish *temporarily* (remember that word), and they do it in a variety of ways. Some coat the wrinkled areas with petrolatum so that when light hits the area, its reflection disguises wrinkles. Some products say they have collagen in them, but this is an animal product, not the same as the collagen in your skin. It coats the skin, and as it dries it tightens it, slightly smoothing out wrinkles. Other creams, containing humectants, plump up the cells to puff out small wrinkles by trapping moisture in the epidermis. Still others contain chemicals called mucopolysaccharides which soak up moisture and smooth the skin. All may "work" in that they temporarily improve appearance. But it doesn't last.

A number of new antiaging products do seem to cause new cell growth, but they do so by causing a harmless inflammation that fools the skin into reacting as if you had an injury. The new cells just move to the surface a little faster (when I say a little, I mean a little; eleven days instead of the normal fifteen), but they don't arrest the breakdown of collagen and elastin in the dermis, so aging still continues and wrinkles keep coming.

People are always looking for ways to stay young-looking, so manufacturers keep coming up with more exotic and expensive products. But you know what? The best advice is to stay out of the sun, or wear a sunscreen or block when you do go out in it. If you don't want to give up your tan, see a plastic surgeon.

• *WRINKLES AWAY* •

Skin renews itself approximately every four weeks. Nutrition affects skin tone and color, so it's essential that you feed yourself properly. Dieting affects your skin tone, as do frequent, rapid weight losses and gains, which will make your skin sag. When you put on weight, the extra fat fills in wrinkles, but a loss that occurs faster than your skin's elasticity can accommodate will leave you with saggy skin.

You can also avoid getting wrinkles in your face by sleeping on your back. Folding and creasing your face for hours every night can cause lines to form, or so I'm told. In general, try to do as much as you can to protect your skin; you can inherit skin that wrinkles prematurely, but you can't blame your ancestors for the wrinkles you get from not taking care of your skin.

On the other hand, no matter what kind of skin we inherit and how well we take care of it, Mom Nature and Pop Time have their own timetables. In your twenties you can expect to see fine lines around your eyes and maybe a few forehead lines. Those lines get a little deeper in your thirties, and a few laugh lines are bound to sprout around your nose and lips. In your forties, tissue sags a little more, and all the lines get deeper.

If the above is enough to make your whole body sag and wrinkle up, well, take heart. Mom Nature compensates for those ten-year changes. If all goes well, each decade brings new self-confidence, making life easier and more fun.

And if you keep your sense of humor, those wrinkles will mostly be smile lines. What's that quote? You live with the face you were born with until middle age, and then you have the face you deserve. So, think happy and you'll be happy. Think about all the glamorous over-forty women who are media stars. Middle age is "in" and getting more "in" as the baby-boom generation ages.

• *SUMMER SUN* •

So, you still want to be a burnt offering by worshiping the sun incorrectly. Well, getting a sunburn is the least of your worries. Not only does the sun age skin, leaving it leathery—it has been linked to several forms of cancer.

If you don't believe all the dermatologists, cosmetologists, and smart, young-looking older women, look around you wherever sun-bathers gather. Look for a person who's twenty-five to thirty years old and who tans every year, and then look for a person who's forty to fifty years old, who's been in the sun a lot. Compare the backs of their necks to the skin about two or three inches down their backs.

You will see a remarkable difference between the two sections of skin.

Where I live in southern Texas, if you stand outside at high noon in June, July, or August and let your skin absorb only ten minutes of ultraviolet rays, you will still get a slight burn. I turn pink walking down the road to my mailbox!

For those of you who insist on broiling yourselves, consider this: the Food and Drug Administration rates the sun-protection factors (SPF) in products that block or screen the sun's harmful rays, and these gradations are printed on the container.

- *SPF 2 to 4:* the minimum protection, best suited to those lucky souls who rarely burn and usually tan easily and deeply
- *SPF 4 to 6:* moderate protection, for people who tan well
- *SPF 6 to 8:* extra protection, for people who burn moderately and tan only gradually
- *SPF 8 to 14:* maximum protection, for people who usually burn easily and rarely tan well
- *SPF 15 and up:* ultra protection for people who burn easily and never tan. This is what I use.

Most dermatologists say that anything above an eight will give you good protection.

Whatever the SPF factor of your sunscreen or sunblock, it probably comes off easily. So be sure to apply it while sunning and reapply it after you swim. How to apply it? First make sure your skin is clean and dry. Then put on with an even, one-way stroke. Rubbing can peel the lotion off. Don't forget to apply the sunscreens *over* your moisturizer and *under* your makeup. I do this every morning as part of my normal routine.

The chemicals to look for in sun-protection products are titanium dioxide and zinc oxide, these are opaque materials that will *block* the sunlight. Lifeguards usually use products containing these ingredients.

Sun-protection lotions and gels that *absorb* rays include **PABA** (para-aminobenzoic acid) or derivatives, and benzophenones. Use products that contain both **PABA** and benzophenones, and don't forget to put extra coats on your lips, nose, and that very delicate skin around your eyes. If you have dark circles under your eyes, exposure to sun will usually make them worse.

It's especially important to protect your lips with sunblocking creams. Strong sunlight, along with fatigue and tension, can lead to cold sores. If you're concerned about how these creams will make your lips look, there are some available that look like lip gloss.

If you have very dry skin, avoid sun lotions with an alcohol base. And remember that *one* thick coat of oil-based lotion is equal to two coats of quick-drying gel.

Again, remember to test-spot sun lotions before slathering them all over your body. You may be allergic to **PABA**.

And if you think baby oil or coconut oil is going to protect you against sunburn, you're looking for trouble. Research has shown that applying oils to skin causes a broiling effect. You actually burn faster if you baste yourself with oil while roasting in the sun.

Keep in mind, too, that certain medications make you even more susceptible to sunburn, so if you are taking a medication regularly, ask your doctor about sunbathing before you do it. Among those substances that heighten skin's sensitivity are: barbiturates, water pills, sedatives, antihistamines, blood pressure reducers, and oral contraceptives.

Some studies suggest that drinking diet sodas and washing with deodorant soaps before sunbathing may make certain types of skin more susceptible to sunburn. Perfume can also cause an allergic reaction if worn in the sun, such as a rash or numbing of the skin.

The best rule is to tan gradually. Limit your time in the sun, as described in the "Sunning Schedules" section that follows, and then cover up by slipping on a robe, wearing a wide-brimmed hat, and hiding under a beach umbrella. And remember, a cloudy day does not mean you won't get a sunburn. The sun is there behind the clouds. Reflection by water or snow can double the sun's lethal effect on your skin.

Sunning Schedules

The sun's rays strike the earth at the most direct and skin-damaging angle between the hours of 10:00 A.M. and 2:00 P.M. (11:00 A.M. and 3:00 P.M. daylight time). So do your sunning before or after these most harmful hours. Remember, the sun's radiation becomes more intense the closer you get to the equator, so it can take you half the time to get a sunburn in the tropics. Keep this in mind if you go south for vacation.

A suncreen's SPF (sun-protection factor) numbers are based on the time it takes for skin to show its first pink blush. If your skin, unprotected by any screen or blocker, would turn pink after about twenty-five minutes of minimal erythema dose (MED) of sun, scientists say you have "a MED of twenty-five." If you have a MED of twenty-five, and you apply a product that gives you a protection of six, you probably can stay in the sun six times twenty-five minutes, or two and a half hours—*if* you have followed the instructions on the label (reapplying it after swimming or sweating, etc.).

The following sunning times are based on average MEDs for skin types and proper application of No. 15 SPF products (maximum

Skin Type	Eyes	Hair	Reaction to Sun	MED (min.)	Sun-Protection Product	Time in Sun (min.)
very fair, thin skin	light		burn, freckle	10	No. 15	150
fair	light	dark blond or auburn	tan slowly, burn	15	No. 15	225
medium	light brown	light brown	tan well slowly, burn without sunscreen	20	No. 15	300
olive-yellow	dark	black or dark brown	tan more than burn	30	No. 15	450
light brown	brown	dark	tan well with protection	45	No. 15	675
black	dark	dark	burn without protection	120	No. 15	1800

sun-protection-factor products) under the best conditions, which are: careful application to all exposed skin, no excess sweating, and reapplication (including to those peek-a-boo openings of certain stylish swimsuits).

To figure out the amount of time that you should spend in the sun under ideal conditions, find the description that best suits you, and multiply the MED by the number on your sun-protection product. Take into account such factors as how close you are to the equator, the time of day, and if you are swimming or sweating.

Also, remember that the MEDs given are *averages;* your MED may be more or less. Observe how long it takes for you to show pink when you bask in the sun—and I mean pink, not *red.* It's probably less time than you think. If you're a regular sunbather, you know that many times you don't "feel pink," and in the sunshine you may not think you look pink. But when you finally step inside, you'll see how red your skin is. And you're bound to suffer that night, as you "burn up" instead of sleep!

"Sunburned" Hair

Make a special effort to cover your hair when sunbathing. Not only can the sun burn your scalp, but if your hair is treated or colored, it may change color completely. One good thing about sunbathing is that if you apply oils or conditioners to your hair before sunbathing, the heat helps the oils penetrate.

We all know about the blondes who spritz their hair with diluted lemon juice before sunbathing to heighten those blond streaks. If you bleach your hair this way you have to condition it well afterward. Brunettes can help their hair color along with a rinse of cooled espresso coffee, and redheads can rinse with cooled tea. Always rinse your hair as soon as possible after swimming in salt or chlorinated water—both can dry your hair out.

Sunburn Relief

Even the most careful sunbathers occasionally get sunburned, so here is some advice from Dr. Frederic Haberman, a nationally known dermatologist. If you begin to look pink when you're sitting out in the sun, that pink means red. Get out of the sun and into a cool bath as fast as you can.

FIRST-DEGREE SUNBURN If your skin is red and swollen, and you are in pain, you have a first-degree sunburn. Hydrocortisone creams, sold over the counter, will relieve the pain, as will applying compresses, made either from moist cornstarch or a commercial oatmeal extract (which can also be purchased in drugstores). Sprinkle the powder through a flour sifter into your bathtub as it is filling with cool water, or wrap regular dry oatmeal in a clean, old stocking or cloth bag, then run your bath water through it; afterward, throw away the oatmeal.

You will get some relief from sunburn if you apply moist compresses of water, milk, or witch hazel on burned skin every two to four hours. Ice, ice water, milk, yogurt, witch hazel, cucumber juice or slices, apple slices, and raw potato slices are all kitchen remedies that some people swear by, but I like to use apple cider vinegar. Some folks sprinkle talc on their sheets. Aspirin can help ease the pain and inflammation, but aspirin or aspirin substitutes do not help swelling and redness.

SECOND-DEGREE SUNBURN   This can lead to infection. If your skin is lobster red and breaks out in blisters, you are suffering from a second-degree burn. See your doctor!

Bleach Away a Fading Tan

After summer is all over and you are tired of your fading tan, you can get rid of that muddy look by scrubbing with a loofah or abrasive puff when you take a bath. Add the juice of three lemons to the bath water to bleach out the last vestiges of your hard-earned bronze. Makeup with a hint of mauve will help cover up the yellowish look of a fading tan.

But why, oh why, sit in the sun anyway? Whenever I feel the urge to look like I have a tan, I use one light coat of a quick-tanning product on my legs and arms every few days and a bronze gel on my neck and shoulders.

• *ACNE-PRONE SKIN* •

Doesn't it seem that blemishes always pop up at just the wrong time? Not that there's ever a *right* time. But some times are unquestionably wronger than others—like the night of a big date or your wedding day. On my wedding day three big ones blossomed smack in the middle of my cheek.

Those of you who suffer from severe acne should be treated by a dermatologist. The results can be amazing.

But do the rest of you, who squirm in anguish at the sight of that occasional pimple, know that one-third of women, aged twenty to fifty, have skin that breaks out, at least occasionally? So you are not alone—and acne is *not* just for adolescents.

Your skin breaks out because hormonal changes in your body are causing the oil glands in your skin to get larger, thereby producing more oil. Then your pores are getting clogged by that oil and bacteria, producing blackheads, whiteheads, pimples, and a whole lot of heartache.

A doctor can prescribe antibiotics, such as tetracycline, or various skin treatments to fight the bacteria, and other medications such as vitamin A acid (Retin-A).

The FDA has approved over-the-counter acne medications made with sulfur, sulfur resorcinol, and benzoyl peroxide. But be sure to follow the directions for these products—they are potent. If your skin becomes too dry, use them every other day instead of every day. I like to dot such medications on each blemish individually, rather than coating my entire face.

If you use benzoyl peroxide, be careful. Some of my friends with teens who use it say that it bleaches towels, pillowcases, and the necklines of T-shirts (especially if it's not properly rinsed off). Also, when someone using the product gropes along the walls of the bathroom for a towel, benzoyl peroxide bleaches handprints, leaving a mark.

Most doctors agree that washing your face gently with soap and warm water three to four times a day is the best way to deal with acne. Some recommend using antibacterial soap, followed by astringent applications to remove any remaining oil. Steer away from heavy, oil-based cosmetics in favor of water-based, oil-free products.

Cosmetic Ingredients to Avoid

Research has revealed that certain ingredients in beauty products make acne-prone skin anything but beautiful. In *Your Skin, a Dermatologist's Guide to a Lifetime of Beauty and Health* (Berkley, 1983) dermatologist Frederic Haberman, M.D. and coauthor Denise Fortino list the following cosmetics ingredients, known to cause a variety of adverse reactions:

Isopropyl isostearate, isopropyl palmitate, isopropyl lanolate
Isostearyl neopentanoate
Butylstearate, isocetyl stearate
Octyl stearate, octyl palmitate
Myristyl myristate, PG 2 myristyl propionate
Decyl oleate
Acetol acetulan
Amberate P
Crude coal tar
Lanosterin, Langogene
Sterolan

Acetylated lanolin, ethyloxylated lanolin
D and C red dyes (common in blushers)*

Detergents such as sodium laurel sulfate, hexadecyl alcohol, hexylene glycol, and polyethylene glycol also aggravate acne-prone skin.

One ingredient in many cosmetics that is not on this list is isoprophyl myristate, which penetrates deep into pores and clogs them if skin is acne-prone. This same ingredient can be found in a product used by mechanics to loosen rusty nuts and bolts. Scary, huh? But Dr. Haberman does list some ingredients that are safe for acne-prone skin, such as makeups containing pigments, water, glycerin, alcohol, and propylene glycole.

Be careful. Even makeups that are "dermatologist-tested," "hypoallergenic," or "medicated" can contain some of the ingredients listed above, Dr. Haberman points out in his book. Read labels and test makeup for oil by applying some of the product to a dull-finished paper or brown grocery-sack paper. Leave it on the paper for twelve hours. If you see oil streaks when you examine the paper under a light, don't buy it.

Makeup Isn't the Only Culprit in the Acne Caper

HABITS Do you often lean your chin or cheeks on your hand? (I just caught myself doing this!) Check these areas. Do they have acne? Habits like keeping your hands on your face or picking at your skin unconsciously irritate acne, as will any kind of pressure or friction, such as holding musical instruments, wearing tight sweatbands or other headgear. Shoulder (or bra) straps and even casts and bandages can aggravate acne, too.

OCCUPATIONAL HAZARDS Cooks and mechanics who work around grease often get acne. People who use carbon paper should be careful not to get the carbon on their faces; it, too, can cause your skin to break out.

CLEANLINESS CUE It's a tough problem, but one thing's certain: acne is not, like the old wives' tales say, a sign that you don't keep clean. In fact, overly vigorous "treatments" of scrubbing or

* Frederic Haberman, M.D., and Denise Fortino, *Your Skin* (New York: Jove, 1983), p. 46.

drying can actually cause it. Some of the things you use for your grooming routines can cause acne—coal-tar dyes, dandruff shampoos, hair pomades. Then add steroids, heat, humidity, sunbathing, and insecticides to the list. Although sun seems to improve acne-prone skin temporarily, its aftereffects—thickening of the skin due to tanning—can put a layer of cells on the skin that are hard to slough off and that clog pores and hair follicles. In general, acne-prone skin should be protected from the sun with nongreasy sunscreens.

Foods Can Aggravate Acne

Some foods, such as kelp, spinach, seaweed, and shellfish, which contain iodides and flourides, can make your acne worse. As Dr. Haberman points out in *Your Skin: A Dermatologist's Guide to a Lifetime of Beauty and Health*, if you think a certain food causes your acne to flare up, avoid it for a while and see if your skin clears; then eat it again to see if you break out. If you do, put it on the list of foods to avoid.

   If you find out that iodides in certain foods make you break out, avoid iodized salt. Iodine was added to salt years ago to prevent goiters (enlarged thyroid), but now nutritionists are saying that Americans may have more acne than Europeans because of an iodine overload. Europeans use only one-tenth the iodine in their salt than we do.

Hiding Blemishes

Many products designed to hide acne actually contain some of the ingredients that aggravate it. *Beware! Read those labels!*

   Here's how I cover a blemish: I take the tip or end of an eyeshadow brush or a cotton-tipped swab, tap it into my coverup makeup, then dot it on the blemish. I do this several times, until the blemish is covered. Then I gently tap the spot with a clean finger. Of course, you should cover the blemish *before* you put your makeup on.

• TEST TO FIND OUT YOUR SKIN TYPE •

Is your skin dry, oily, or combination? Find out with the following test.

Wash your face with shaving cream. Rinse. Wait about three hours so that your skin can revert to its regular self. Then take cigarette papers or any other thin tissue paper and press pieces of it on your face. If the paper sticks, your skin is oily. If it doesn't stick, your skin is dry. If the paper sticks on some areas and not others, you probably have combination skin.

• OILY SKIN •

Oily skin is a mixed blessing. It won't wrinkle as early as dry skin, but chances are you'll be acne-prone, even past your teen years. If you have oily skin, you usually have coarse-textured skin with large pores and oily patches that attract dirt, causing makeup to discolor.

The magic age for oily skin is about twenty-five—before then, you usually have excess oil all over your face; later, you may develop combination skin or have excess oil on your "T-zone," across your forehead and down your nose and chin. This, by the way, describes me to a T.

Tips for Oily Skin

Wash often with detergent soap and lukewarm water; rinse *thoroughly* and dry. Use a loofah or wash-up puffs about three times weekly. Follow with astringent to remove remaining oil.

Astringents don't erase large pores, but they do minimize them by causing a minor irritation that puffs up the skin around the pores, thereby making them less noticeable.

When you can't wash your face, blot it with tissues or a clean sponge during the day to remove oil as it accumulates. (I carry one in my makeup bag in my purse.) Dust with powder to freshen makeup. Also, shampoo your hair often. You've got to keep skin clean—and scalp is skin!

Makeup for Oily Skin

Never use heavy or oily base makeup; use water-base or oil-free instead. Water will be first or near the top of the ingredients list. Set makeup by dusting lightly with baby powder or talc. In fact, it's a good idea to dust with talc or baby powder, even when you're not wearing makeup.

Facials for Oily Skin

Don't panic if your face seems excessively oil about two weeks before menstruation; you have lots of company. This is the time to use stronger cleanser and to wash more often. (Masks made with citrus fruits or milk products are good for oily skin.)

Here are some kitchen remedies for oily skin. (When using any of these, be sure to avoid the delicate eye area.)

- *Egg Facial:* beat together one teaspoon each of egg white and milk; add a few drops of honey and lemon juice; apply to face; let dry and rinse off with tepid water.
- *More Egg:* make a paste of two beaten egg whites, one tablespoon nonfat dry milk powder, and one teaspoon honey. Leave on face for twenty minutes; rinse off with lukewarm water.
- *Almond Oatmeal:* apply paste made from a handful of oatmeal or ground almonds and warm water to damp skin; leave on for five to ten minutes; take wet washcloth and wipe off; rinse well with warm water.
- *Yeast:* spread a paste of one pack dry, or one cake brewer's yeast, mixed in warm water on your face; leave on for ten minutes; rinse off.
- *Veggies:* place unpeeled, sliced cucumbers or potatoes on your face for a summer freshener while you rest.
- *Grated Potato Facial:* wrap grated potato (unpeeled) in gauze or cheesecloth; apply to face; cover face with cotton washcloth dipped in milk; leave on twenty minutes; rinse off with lukewarm water.
- *Fruities:* mash one unpeeled pear to smooth paste or whir in blender; add membrane from six grapefruit segments, blend; add a small amount of comfrey tea (from health food store); apply to face; rest ten minutes while you drink the rest of the tea; rinse off with tepid water.
- *Mist:* add one teaspoon table salt to water in a plant mister bottle; spritz-mist face; blot dry with soft towel.
- *Loosen Blackheads:* In *Your Skin: A Dermatologist's Guide to a Lifetime of Beauty and Health,* Dr. Haberman suggests that you pour boiling water into a sink or bowl; add herbs of choice—chamomile or comfrey are my favorites—and then hold your face about twelve

inches from the water for five to ten minutes, while you tent a towel over your head to keep in the steam. Dry face with soft towel.

These steaming and facial scrubs work wonders keeping blackheads away. The trick is to keep dead skin, dirt, and oil from accumulating and clogging pores.

For a quick and easy steamer, I heat a wet towel in the microwave oven, then tent it on my face. Be sure it's not too hot when you remove it from the microwave; you want to steam your face—not burn it.

• DRY SKIN •

So your skin feels like it's too tight; like it's so dry that if you smile your face will crack. Well, dry facial skin needs moisturizers the way chapped hands need lotions; but don't load up on heavy, greasy products or all you'll get is clogged pores. Many dermatologists say dry skin needs water, not oil, and that the best bet is to keep moisture in your skin by applying lotions to seal it in while your skin is still damp.

Mild soaps without perfume are kindest to dry skin. Before you wash, remove makeup with diluted (cq) alcohol or witch hazel; rinse and wash. Dry skin's flakiness and crepiness are as much a problem as oily skin's greasy shine. Also, harsh weather will chap dry skin and make you miserable.

Climate Conditions

I was really surprised to learn about the different ways the climate affects skin products. For example, most moisturizers and creams contain glycerin and glycote combinations called humectants. In damp weather, these humectants draw moisture from the air into your skin; but when the air is dry, humectants are said to draw water out of your skin and put it into the air. So, the advice from beauty experts is: in damp weather or climates, use moisturizers; in dry, desert heat, seal the moisture in your skin with oils. Dermatologists agree that even people who are sensitive to oils can usually use mineral oil or petroleum jelly without breaking out. Personally, I prefer mineral oil to moisturize my skin.

Makeup for Dry Skin

Use cream or oil-base makeup and blusher to avoid the dull look of dry skin. You can get a moist, dewy look by thinning out your makeup with a dab of moisturizer and a few drops of water. Just mix it in your palm. Use translucent powder; dust on with a brush; and remove excess with a clean brush or cotton ball. Some people like to dab at their skins with a damp cosmetic sponge after putting on their makeup.

Dry Skin Facials

Apply all with gentle circular motion, *always* avoiding the delicate eye area. Remember, if you continually have flaky skin or flaky patches of skin in spite of all your tender loving care, see your doctor. You may have a skin or nutritional problem.

• *Banana Facial:* blend one teaspoon each of yogurt and egg yolk; add dab of mashed banana; pat on face; leave on fifteen minutes, or until it dries; remove with warm, then cool water.

• *Banana Honey:* mash one medium banana; add one tablespoon honey; smooth on face; leave on fifteen minutes; rinse with warm water.

• *Banana Cream:* mix one small, ripe, mashed banana with two tablespoons of sour cream and one teaspoon honey; leave on fifteen minutes; rinse with warm water.

• *Eggy Facial:* one part egg to two parts yogurt; follow same directions as banana facial.

• *Egg Honey:* mix one tablespoon honey and one egg yolk; leave on fifteen minutes; rinse off with tepid water. If this seems too gooey, add a few drops of water. And don't forget to apply it to your neck.

• *Egg Oil:* combine one egg yolk mixed with one teaspoon each of honey and sweet almond oil (or cream); smooth on face and throat; leave on ten to fifteen minutes; rinse with warm water.

• *Other Eggies:* mix an egg yolk with a mashed avocado or a mashed, pared peach and wheat germ oil; leave on fifteen minutes; rinse.

• *Dairy:* mix equal parts of yogurt and buttermilk; pat on face, neck, and throat; let dry; rinse with cool or tepid water.

• *Dairy Cream for Extradry Skin:* let buttermilk stand overnight at room temperature; skim off the cream that has risen to the top and pat it on face, neck, and throat; let dry; rinse off with cool or tepid water.

• *Witch Hazel Mask:* blend one teaspoon of boric acid and two tablespoons dry powdered milk with enough witch hazel to make a paste; apply to neck and face (avoid eye area); let dry; wash off with mild soap and water; apply witch hazel as an astringent and a moisturizer.

• *Easy Treatment:* warm petroleum jelly by placing jar in warm water; apply to clean face; dip hand towel in warm water; wring out water; place towel on face and leave on for few minutes; remove petroleum jelly with tissue or cloth; rinse well with warm water. This facial is especially good for itchy, dry skin or skin that's been exposed to harsh weather. (While you're applying the petroleum jelly to your face don't forget your neck; let it soothe and smooth your hands and elbows at the same time.)

• *NORMAL SKIN* •

Here's the good news for those of you who are tired of reading about oily, dry, and sensitive skins: dermatologists agree that hardly *any-one* has "normal" skin.

Normal skin is firm, has an even texture, an equal balance of oil and moisture, very few blemishes, and a natural color with a clear, well-scrubbed look. And it tans instead of burns.

Did I just describe the girl with the long blond hair and perfect legs who sat next to you in your freshman high school English class —that same year even your acne had acne? Don't we all remember the Nancy Nices who made us feel like Kitty Klutzes? I had acne in high school, so I know what it's like when the only regular date you have is once a month—at the dermatologist's office.

Well, my research for this book has taught me that even Nancy Nice loses the moisture in her skin after she passes forty or so. And people with normal skin can begin to show dry patches when they are only twenty-five, after which they develop the most common skin type of all—combination skin.

• *COMBINATION SKIN* •

If you have dry areas and oily spots, you have what's called combination skin. The oily spots usually hit your T-zone, around your forehead, nose, and chin. The oily areas may have large pores and break out frequently; the dry areas will have finer pores and show wrinkles prematurely.

The trick is to treat each area appropriately. It may seem like a bother, but doing so will give your skin the most balanced look possible. You can protect the dry areas of your face with petroleum jelly while you steam your face to cleanse the pores in the oily areas. When you cleanse your skin, be sure to pay special attention to the oily areas with chilled astringents and to the dry patches with moisturizers.

Normal and Combination Skin Facials

You can use separate facial mixes for the dry and oily parts of combination skin, or you can look for facials that contain a combination of ingredients appropriate for oily and dry skin.

Normal skin usually needs no special care. (That must be lovely!) Most experts say facials aren't really necessary until you hit forty or so—unless, that is, normal skin suddenly stops being normal.

The following facials, recommended for normal or combination skin by Dr. Haberman in *Your Skin: A Dermatologist's Guide to a Lifetime of Beauty and Health,* by a nationally known dermatologist, are for normal or combination skin. Remember, never apply them to the delicate eye area.

• *Apples and Honey:* in a blender, whir up one medium apple, one tablespoon each of honey and skim milk; apply to skin; leave on twenty minutes; wash off with warm water.

• *Lemon and Honey:* dissolve three tablespoons of honey in two tablespoons boiling water; make a paste by adding and mixing in two tablespoons lemon juice; cool to lukewarm; apply; leave on for twenty minutes; wash off with lukewarm water.

• *Lemon and Apricot:* blend one teaspoon apricot oil with two beaten egg yolks; add one teaspoon lemon juice; mix well; apply; leave on twenty minutes; wash off with lukewarm water.

• *Almond and Witch Hazel:* make a paste with a third cup of ground almonds and enough witch hazel to moisten; apply; leave on for fifteen minutes; wash off in warm water.

• *Strawberry and Butter:* mash about ten large strawberries and add one teaspoon each of butter and lemon juice; apply; leave on for about ten to fifteen minutes; rinse off with warm water.

• *Egg White Plus:* beat one egg white until frothy; add one of the following ingredients—one teaspoon of lemon juice, or about a teaspoon of apple cider vinegar, or two teaspoons lime juice and a drop of honey; apply; let dry; rinse off with wet washcloth.

• *Apple and Wine:* blend the pulp of one small apple with two tablespoons ground almonds and enough white wine to make a paste. Cleanse face with half of mixture; wash off; apply second half to face as mask; leave on ten to fifteen minutes; wash off with warm water.

• *Peanut Butter and Honey:* don't eat it—apply it! This is for normal or dry skin. Mix two parts honey to three parts smooth peanut butter; rub on with circular motion for cleanser; rinse off well.

• *Veggie:* mash one cooked carrot and half an avocado and mix with three tablespoons of yogurt and about a tablespoon of minced parsley; let mixture rest at room temperature for several minutes before applying to face; leave on about fifteen minutes; wash off with warm water.

• *BLACK SKIN* •

Black skin, whether it's oily, dry, or combination, comes with its own set of problems. Older black skin can lose pigment the way older white skin can get pigmentation brown spots, as well as from rashes or acne or scars. Black skin may also be more susceptible to keloids, those raised scars that are the result of infections or acne. Many dermatologists suggest that black skin should be treated with milk products to avoid such irritations. They also warn that black-skinned people with acne must be cautious about using benzoyl peroxide products. Why? Benzoyl peroxide easily penetrates darker skin and may actually darken treated areas. Vitamin A preparations for acne tend to lighten black skin. To be safe, black-skinned people should consult with a dermatologist before attempting to use either type of product even if the resultant skin discolorations are only temporary. Your doctor can prescribe mild products and treatments that will help acne *without* harming your skin.

• *SENSITIVE SKIN* •

We all know someone who seems to break out in a rash at the mere mention of wool sweaters, plants that aren't even in the poison ivy category, or beauty products that everyone else seems to use with no problems.

Whatever your skin type, you can develop allergies and sensitivities—with resulting skin blotches, hives, swelling, itching, and dilated blood vessels—to just about anything. You can even become allergic to those old-faithful products you've been using for years (sometimes it may seem to happen overnight).

If you are allergic to foods, plants, or other irritants, the best advice anyone can give you is to avoid known troublemakers. Stick with products that are formulated without such irritants as detergents, scents, dyes, lanolin, and formaldehyde. Use soft washcloths. And remember that hot, spicy foods, coffee, and alcohol can cause dilated blood vessels in your skin. And a ruddy nose only looks good on Rudolph the red-nosed reindeer.

According to some beauty experts, facials containing aloe vera, chamomile, rose hips, azulene, wheat germ oil, allantoin, collagen, and panthenol can minimize broken capillaries in the face. A dermatologist can treat them more permanently with a special procedure called electrodisiccation.

Too much exposure to cold, wind, or sun harms sensitive skin. Other known irritants are hair sprays, deodorants, hair dyes, bath crystals, nail polish, depilatories, bronzers, colognes, and aftershaves.

Teatime Skin Soothers

Chamomile tea is a favorite remedy for skin irritated by sun, food, or drink. Some people brew up a batch of tea, cool it, and apply it to the face or other irritated areas. As a bonus, they take a relaxation break and drink the rest of the tea.

Any kind of tea is a skin soother. Steep two tea bags in one cup of boiling water; allow to cool to room temperature. Using the tea bags as sponges, pat your face with the tea, dipping the bags into it frequently for five minutes. Blot skin dry. Since less expensive teas contain the most tannic acid, and the tannic acid is soothing to your skin, the cheaper the tea, the better.

Itchy Skin Soothers

Here are some remedies for itchy skin, suggested by dermatologists:

- Apply moistened, crushed aspirin to the swollen area.
- Apply ice or cold compresses.
- Dust cornstarch over oozing rashes.
- Apply watery paste of oatmeal or baking soda to affected areas.
- Apply paste of unflavored meat tenderizer—who needs to smell like "barbecue" or "garlic"?—to bites and stings.
- Apply calamine lotion to affected areas.
- Apply sap of aloe vera leaf. Break the leaf to start the sap running and apply directly. Recent research at the University of Texas Health Science Center in San Antonio has shown that aloe plants are useful in treating skin problems only when applied fresh. According to researchers, processed aloe juices for salves and so forth are of no value—not good news for people who process the plant and swear by their products!
- Prevent heat rash by dusting your skin with talc or other powder.
- Prevent rashes from metal jewelry by painting your jewelry with clear nail polish.

Poison Ivy

Remember, you don't have to touch poison ivy to get a rash. You can develop an adverse reaction to poison ivy by touching things that have been in contact with the plant—bike tires that have ridden through it or a dog or cat that's walked through it. If you wash the area after you've been exposed to the poison ivy oils, chances are the itchy, burning rash won't appear. Rinse first with water, then wash well with soap (some people recommend brown laundry soap, but any good, pure soap will do), or take a shower. After washing with soap and water, rinse well, remembering to clean under your fingernails. Take everything into account—whatever clothing came in contact with the plant, etc. You should of course shampoo your pet if he came into contact with poison ivy. Be sure to wear rubber gloves while doing this.

If you are too late with preventives, here are some ways to relieve the miseries. For a mild case, apply cloths soaked in saltwater (one teaspoon salt to one pint tepid water) or diluted boric acid to the afflicted areas. Ice water, milk, calamine lotion, or a tepid bath can give relief for mild cases.

And keep this in mind: a simple case of poison ivy *can* build into a big infection. If your reaction is more than mild, see your doctor!

• TENDER, LOVING CARE HELPS NORMAL OR AVERAGE SKIN •

Even if you don't have problem skin, it's essential that you cleanse and care for your skin properly. One of the biggest mistakes women make is that they use too heavy a hand when applying makeup or taking it off. If you don't give your skin tender, loving care with smooth, gentle strokes, the connective tissues will break down and before you know it you'll have—you guessed it—wrinkles.

Avoid Extremes

Exposing skin to extreme hot or cold can break down the capillaries.

And remember, when you're hiking outdoors in the wintertime, bright red cheeks don't necessarily mean you're the picture of health—especially if the red is surrounded by snow white. This could be an early sign of frostbite!

If you spend a lot of time outdoors in winter, protect your skin with moisturizers and wear wool mufflers or ski masks. Don't forget to apply a sunblock. Winter sun—reflected by snow—is no kinder to your skin than summer sun! Especially in cold weather, using body lotion is crucial. Indoor heating drys your skin. And while we're on the subject of drying, air conditioning and the "processed" air in airplanes will also leave your skin parched. *Moisturize!* You'll be glad you did.

• MOISTURIZING SKIN •

Finding the moisturizer that is best for you isn't easy. All those different labels are terribly confusing. Here's what I've learned about moisturizers.

Most are mixtures of oil and water, with another substance added to keep the oil and water from separating. When there is more water than oil you have a lotion. When there is more oil than water, you have a cream. That's why lotions are better for oily skin and creams are better for dry skin—unless you have certain specific skin problems.

How Moisturizers Work

Moisturizers work by trapping the moisture left on your skin with thin layers of grease or oil. The oil or grease plumps up the cells of your skin with the moisture, thereby protecting it from drying out and wrinkling.

Some of the ingredients you'll find in commercial moisturizers are: petroleum jelly and lanolin (the two heaviest moisturizers and the best for superprotection), mineral oil, urea, stearic or lactic acid, and squalene (derived from shark liver oil). Urea, lactic acid, and squalene are among the substances that are also found in human skin and sweat. Although lanolin is a very good moisturizing oil, I don't suggest you use it if you are acne-prone—it often causes blemish breakouts.

Petroleum jelly is a good heavy-duty moisturizer that is compatible with most skin types. Many women apply olive oil to their faces while they shower or soak in the tub.

Water

Did you know that water is the best moisturizer? Inside and out, it is one of your skin's best friends. Many dermatologists recommend drinking five to six glasses daily to moisturize skin from the inside. And it doesn't have to be that fancy bottled stuff—plain old tap water does the job. Talk about bargains!

It's a good idea to keep the atmosphere in which you live as moist as possible. This doesn't mean you have to buy an expensive humidifier (some newer furnaces have humidifiers built in). You can permeate the air of your home with five to six gallons of water by simmering an eight-quart pot of water on your stove for twenty-four hours. (Add some fragrant cinnamon or a potpourri for a yummy-smelling house! Or you can place pretty containers of water around the house (remember to keep them full); the water will evaporate into the air.

Plant Power

Greenery adds moisture to the air too. Plants that like lots of water and grow fast are the best—ferns, bamboo, begonias, zebra plants, coleus, and others. Keep the soil moist with frequent waterings and mistings. Putting the pots in a shallow tray filled with pebbles or moss and water also helps keep moisture in the air.

Spritzing Plants and Skin

Most beauty experts agree that you should periodically spritz your face during the day with water from a plant mister. Why not do it right after you spritz your plants! Or dab water on your face with cotton balls or makeup squares? When I spend a lot of time on airplanes, I dab or spritz my face regularly.

Drying from Laundry Soap

Using too much laundry detergent in your clothing and bedding can also dry your skin because it tends to remain in fabrics even after the rinse cycle. In the winter, use only about one-fourth the amount of detergent suggested by the manufacturer. Enzyme detergents, powdered bleaches, and whiteners can be powerful irritants. In the summer, always rinse off chlorine or salt after you swim.

Moisturizing at Home

Here's a way to moisturize skin while working in the kitchen: steam your face over the open dishwasher door. But be careful—the steam can get pretty hot. How's this for a hint: save energy *and* put moisture into your home by letting your dishes air dry in the dishwasher after the wash and rinse cycles while steaming your face.

After you've taken steps to add moisture to the atmosphere in your home, don't blow it by overheating. Try to lower the temperature while you sleep—cool air is not as dry as hot air.

Remember:

* Clean skin properly, according to type.
* Remove dead skin cells with washcloths, puffs, or scrubs.
* Apply moisturizers immediately after washing your face to prevent the surface water from evaporating.
* Replenish moisture during the day.

If, after following this advice, you still have problems, see your dermatologist.

• *SKIN PIGMENTATION* •

Melasma

Melasma is the name for those darkened skin areas under the eyes, across the nose, and elsewhere that are often associated with pregnancy or taking birth control pills. These dark areas can be lightened with hydroquinone cream or lotion, which is available in drugstores. But be careful: when you are using bleaching creams stay out of the sun. You can damage your skin. In fact, if you have melasma you should stay out of the sun anyway—it makes discoloration worse.

Bleaching Skin

Using lemon juice as a skin bleach is a practice that goes back to the ancient Greeks. Leave it on whatever areas you want bleached —hands, elbows, knees—for about fifteen minutes.

Vitiligo

Vitiligo is the term for a sudden loss of pigment from patches of any size or shape on any part of the body. Patches of hair can also lose color. Why does this happen? Sometimes, when there has been an injury, the pigment-producing cells may leave an area. And vitiligo can be exacerbated by sunburn, infection, illness, even emotional problems. Exactly *why* some people lose skin or hair pigment is still not known, but research continues.

Repigmentation therapy *is* available, but it is not entirely successful for everyone. It works best for children or young adults, especially if they've had vitiligo less than five years. The therapy, which is time-consuming and must be done under a doctor's supervision, involves medication and exposure to sunlight. Those who are sensitive or allergic to sunlight are not eligible for treatment.

• *MASKS ARE MARVELOUS* •

Some people think masks are of little benefit to your face, and others swear by them. Many dermatologists say that masks *can* improve circulation, tone, remove surface oil, dirt, and dead skin cells, as well as makeup from the skin. After removing a mask, if the mask does not contain a moisturizing agent, you should moisturize.

Aside from its beneficial effects, many people say a facial is a relaxing way to pamper yourself. I couldn't agree more.

Regular salon facials can be expensive, but there are many home remedies you can try that not only make your skin feel good, but are fun to concoct. The following facials can be used on most skin types, but be sure to apply them to clean skin and avoid the eye area.

Heloise Honey Facial

My favorite facial cleanses as well as moisturizes. After cleaning and steaming my face, I apply honey. Then I leave it on for two or three minutes (some people like to leave it on for ten minutes)—until it's sticky. (If you don't believe that honey gets stickier than it was when you applied it, just wait a few minutes.) Then I press in and snap out my fingers on my face—gently! I always avoid the areas around my eyes. Remove honey with a warm, wet towel or washcloth.

For heaven's sake, avoid wearing fuzzy sweaters or similar clothing when using this facial. One of my friends gave herself a Heloise honey facial while wearing an angora sweater and then decided to take off the sweater while her face was still covered with honey. By the time she'd pulled the sweater over her face, she looked like she was trying to grow a beard!

You'll find honey cleans out pores so that they seem to shrink and become smaller, and it really can get rid of blackheads. They sure keep my face clean and smooth. And honey is a bargain—right there in your kitchen.

VARIATIONS ON HONEY FACIALS Mix a teaspoon of honey with six tablespoons water, two tablespoons each of ground orange peel and vinegar, and you have a kitchen-made cleanser for any type of skin.

Or mix one whole fresh egg with enough honey to make a paste; spread paste on face; let harden to mask; rinse with warm water until all the paste is off; rinse with cold water to refresh skin.

Skin Toner

Get our your blender. Whir up the juice of one whole lemon, one-half teaspoon wheat germ oil (from health food store), one-half cup mineral water, and two ice cubes. Apply to clean skin with a cotton ball. Store in the fridge.

Nutty Cleanser

This is a nutty cleanser/skin smoother. Mix almond meal and witch hazel to make a paste; apply to face, scrub gently, avoiding eye area; leave on skin for twenty minutes; rinse off with tepid water. This may look really messy, but it cleans pores and skin surfaces.

Apricot Facial

How about a facial you'll be tempted to drink? Soak twelve dried apricots in boiled water; cover; let soak overnight. Next day, put the apricots into your blender with ten seedless grapes; purée. Sprinkle powdered milk into purée to thicken, and spread mixture on face and neck; let set twelve to fifteen minutes. Rinse with warm water.

An Eggsactly Right Mask

Beat the whites of two eggs to a froth; spread over clean face and throat, avoiding eye area. Let mask dry; rinse with cool water. Used this way, egg whites tighten pores.

Milk of Magnesia Mask

Wash face and neck, then spread on milk of magnesia, avoiding eye area; leave on for fifteen minutes. Apply more milk of magnesia, then wipe with washcloth and warm water. Follow with thorough rinse with tepid water and application of warm olive oil on cotton ball. Leave oil on for five minutes and blot up excess. Milk of magnesia is also good to dab on blemishes. A doctor friend told me that some hospitals use milk of magnesia on bedsores. You'd be surprised by the versatility of certain products. I even use toothpaste to dry up blemishes when I'm on the road.

More Food for Your Face

After cleansing, apply a mask made from equal parts of buttermilk and yogurt; pat paste on face, throat, shoulders, and hands, avoiding eye area; let dry. Rinse off with cool water.

Neck and Chin

Don't forget your neck and the underchin area. The skin on your neck is delicate and wrinkles as easily as your face, so cleanse and *moisturize* it. And, since your neck has no oil glands, remember it needs more special care, such as tightening agents, along with moisturizers.

Throat Cream

Here's a throat cream you can make yourself. Add one-fourth teaspoon alum to an eight-ounce jar of cold cream. (Alum is a tightening agent, and, yes, it's the stuff that makes your canned pickles firm.) You can also use this homemade tightening cream on your breasts for a home-style "European" treatment.

As you massage cream on your neck, use gentle upward and outward movements.

Skin Peel

For a skin peel that works with most skin types, add one tablespoon salt (some like to use sea salt) to one cup hot, but not boiling, water. Allow it to cool a little and then rub gently over wrinkled areas around the mouth, chin, and throat. Avoid the eye area.

Super Cream

In an enamel or pyrex double boiler, melt together three tablespoons each of cocoa butter, sesame oil, lanolin, two tablespoons olive oil, and one tablespoon safflower oil over simmering water. Stir occasionally to blend ingredients well. Add chamomile if you wish. After all ingredients are smoothly blended, remove from heat; cool; apply.

Minty Freshener

Simmer a tablespoon of mint in one cup of milk over low flame—
no bubbling—for five minutes. Turn off flame, put pot aside and
steep, covered, for about an hour. Strain out mint, and add two
tablespoons of honey, stirring and blending well. Sound almost
good enough to eat? Well, put it on your face instead.

Veggie Fresheners

These skin fresheners are good for most skins. Slice cold cucumbers, place slices on your eyelids before you nap. Or slice juicy raw
tomatoes and arrange them on your face while you rest for about
fifteen minutes. Really refreshing!

Facial Steamer

Many experts believe that facials work best if your skin is steamed
before you begin. You don't need a facial steamer; just pour hot
water into a basin, tent a towel over your head, and hold your face
over the water for no more than five minutes. Another way to steam
your face is to apply a washcloth dipped in hot water to your face,
dipping and redipping for about five minutes. Or heat your damp
washcloth in the microwave. Test before using to make sure it's not
too hot.

Your skin will tell you how often a treatment is needed. If your
skin gets sore and dry, you are rubbing too hard and taking treatments too often. Generally, dry skin can use treatment about once
a week or every two weeks for very dry skin; oily skin needs treatment more often. Combination skin can be treated once a week on
the dryer areas and perhaps three times a week on the oily areas.
As always, remoisturize after each treatment.

• BEAUTY BATHING •

I always knew homemade bath aids were popular, but until I went
on a fact-finding mission for this book, I had no idea how many
ways people bathed, soaked, and relaxed. Read on and let some of
the following ideas soak in.

Tub-time Facial

Many people use tub time to nourish their faces as well—the warm misty bath atmosphere helps face creams penetrate better. You can also wring out a washcloth and drape it on your face while you soak, to put some extra moisture into your skin.

Cushiony Comfort

Make a bath pillow with a hot water bottle filled with warm water or roll up a big bath towel and seal it inside a plastic bag. You don't need to buy a special pillow that costs extra money.

Temperature and Timing Count

Water that's too hot or a soak that's too long will take too much oil out of your skin, especially in the winter, when your skin is parched anyway. You don't have to stay in until your skin cells swell up with water and you look like a prune. Generally water temperatures of 85 or 90 degrees are considered tepid, 90 to 100 degrees are warm, and anything above that is considered trouble for your skin.

Soothing Soak

About the only time you should use hot water is to soothe sore muscles. When I've had one of *those* days—you know the kind I mean, when your neck and shoulder muscles are so tight that you're all hunched up like a football player—I fill my tub with hot water, get the thickest bath towel I can find, toss it into the water, and then hop in after it. I keep dipping and dunking that towel in the water and wrapping it around my neck and shoulders until the muscles relax. You can also rub the towel back and forth across your shoulders. Oh, does it feel good!

A Good Soak

For a good soak, stay in the water just long enough to soften dead skin (on your feet, elbows, or elsewhere) so that you can rub it off with a pumice stone, loofah, or abrasive puff. People seem divided on pumice—some think it's too abrasive and rub the wet pumice-stone in soap to soften it. I think it's a question of how your skin feels. Don't give yourself such a vigorous treatment that you make your skin sore, but do get rid of dry, dead skin.

Oil in Bath Water

Some people never bathe without putting oil in the water first; others like to soak five to twenty minutes to open their pores, and then add oil. Whatever you do, be careful when putting oil in the tub or slathering it on your body before showering. Oil is slippery on the tub floor! And you don't want the world's softest skin wrapped in a body cast, do you?

Many beauty consultants suggest slathering on oil *before* going into the bath, and that the best time to put on body lotion or oil is right after your bath or shower, while your skin is still moist. (Pat, don't rub off, water after bathing.) They say the purpose of the lotion or oil is to *seal moisture* in your skin. Petroleum jelly is recommended as a sealant. Put it in the palms of your hands, rub them together, and then rub the jelly all over your body. You may, however, prefer a thinner moisturizer. In that case, use baby oil or mineral oil.

However you bathe, don't bathe more than once a day in the wintertime. In fact, people with very dry skin may have to limit themselves to only three baths a week, with sponge baths in between, to keep skin from getting too dry in winter. Since underarm odor is caused by bacterial action, people who can't bathe as often as necessary can rub alcohol on their underarm areas—it's a great antiseptic and will kill odor-causing bacteria.

After a morning bath, it's better to apply lotion; save heavy creams and oils for evening baths and bedtime beauty. Why? Lotions tend to be lighter and therefore easier on clothing. Heavy-duty moisturizers are those that contain the most petrolatum and mineral oil. Read labels to find out which lotions, creams, or baby products are the heaviest. Petrolatum or mineral oil will usually be listed first, or near the head of the list of ingredients.

Betcha Never Heard of So Many Bath Beautifiers

When it comes to bathing beauty, every woman has her own favorite formula. Consider these.

MILK MAGIC Swirl a package of powdered nonfat dry milk or a quart of regular low-fat (more expensive, though) into a tubful of warm water and soak. This is one of several ways to soothe sunburn as well as yourself. It's been said that Marie Antoinette bathed in milk, but don't lose your head over the idea! (Sorry—couldn't resist.)

SEA SALT SPECIAL For a super cleansing bath, add a half pound of sea salt to warm water. Some people who like to exercise in the tub say the salt gives you the buoyancy of being in the ocean or the Great Salt Lake in Utah. I haven't tried this one yet, but it sounds good.

FRAGRANCE FIX Save those sample vials of perfume that you get from department stores and add them to a couple of capfuls of baby oil for a scentsational soak. You can also add leftover perfume to the water or rinse out an empty perfume bottle in your bath to get every last smidgen of scent. Some people like to mix up their own bath oil, using perfume and coconut or almond or other oil.

CIDER SOOTHER Apple cider vinegar—about two cupfuls to a tub—is good for a soothing bath, especially for sunburn, itchy skin problems such as poison ivy, or any time you're tired and need a lift. Some people pour the vinegar into the water; others prefer to splash it on their bodies *before* sitting down in the water.

OATMEAL BATH Oatmeal, either au naturel or in a bag, is another good skin soother for the bath. Some people dangle a cloth bag of oatmeal (two cups or so) on the faucet as the tub fills and then rub their skin with the bag after it's moistened by the water flow. Others use this as a sunburn soother. Just add the oatmeal to the water, soak in it, and then apply heavy cream to wet skin, followed by the application of a half yogurt–half buttermilk mixture. Sounds almost nutritious (and maybe fattening) doesn't it?

HERBAL CHOICES A variety of herbs, alone or in combination, can be put into a cloth or net bag and tossed into the tub or hung on the faucet as the tub fills to soothe skin and make your bath smell good. Here are some of them: rosemary, chamomile, any variety of mint, comfrey, rose petals, lavender, yarrow, or camphor. You can also steam your face with the herbs and then toss the bag into your bath to use every bit of their "flavor." About a half cup of dry or fresh herbs will do the job, depending on how much flavor you want.

Caution: If your allergies are triggered by plants, do a spot test, as described in Chapter 1, "Strictly Personal." first. If you have allergies, the herbs may send you right into a milk or vinegar bath, and you'll *never* get out of your kitchen or tub.

• SHAVING RITES •

Have you ever wondered why we shave our legs instead of our arms —which are, after all, more visible? Well, I still haven't figured that one out.

But illogic aside, now that the protest years of the sixties and seventies are behind us, smooth legs are back in. So, unless you cheat by wearing slacks or boots, chances are leg shaving is part of your beauty routine.

Now that we've moved into the eighties, another old wives' tale has bitten the dust: the idea that shaving causes hair to grow back thicker and/or darker. Any dermatologist will tell you that, although the hair may look thicker and/or darker because you got accustomed to the look of bare skin (or maybe it was getting darker anyway), it wasn't *shaving* that caused the change. So, now that we've dispensed with that myth, here are some hints on hair removal.

Leg Shaving

Before shaving sensitive skin, smooth on olive oil or moisturing cream; work up a good lather with soap or shaving cream to prevent nicks; shave, and then apply moisturizer.

I like to shave my legs in the shower. I usually use whatever men's shaving cream is on sale, or the cheapest brand. Once, I picked up a can of menthol. It was so good and tingly that I tried some on my face—it felt like I'd just had a facial! Now part of my beauty/shower routine is to pat some of that good old menthol on my face. I leave it on while I bathe, and when I've rinsed it all off, I feel like smiling all day. Maybe that's why men look so good after they shave—because they feel so perked up by their shaving creams. Well, if so, we've got their secret now, haven't we?

Baby lotion or other body/hand lotions are good substitutes for shaving cream, although some hand lotions with a high alcohol content will wake up your skin too much!

And don't forget, if you find yourself in the shower, dripping wet, without any shaving cream, you can work up a good lather with bar soap (not great but adequate), shampoo, or cream rinse.

If your legs are polka-dotted or look like they have the measles, you are probably shaving too closely and/or in the wrong direction. Shaving against the grain (the direction in which the hairs grow) can result in the hair growing back trapped in the skin, which in turn causes inflammation of the hair follicle.

Shaving Underarms

When, after shaving your underarms, you apply certain deodorants, your skin may become irritated. Play it safe. Shave underarms at night, pat on mild witch hazel to close pores, then let your skin rest overnight *before* using a deodorant.

Other Ways to Remove Hair

Some women say that though the shave isn't as close, electric shavers are kinder to their sensitive skin. Maybe it's because the shave isn't so close that the irritation is less. If you have a problem with shaving, you may want to consider an electric shaver.

Bleaching and depilatory lotions and creams disguise or get rid of unwanted hair. But be sure to always follow the directions and take a patch test first with any of these just to make sure you're not allergic.

Waxing is another effective method of hair removal that works best if you have about three weeks' worth of hair growth. Sun and sweat irritate newly waxed skin, so beware of sunbathing or vigorous outdoor sports the day after waxing.

There are plenty of beauty routines that need special scheduling. Listen to this horror story. One of my friends waxed the mustache on her upper lip just before a big date. Afterward, she applied her makeup as usual. Some hours later, as she and her VIF (very important fellow) were having a romantic dinner in a fancy restaurant, she began to feel a burning sensation on her lip—and it wasn't a kiss. When she went to the rest room to check, she discovered a "mustache" of red skin right where she'd used the wax!

She has since learned to plan ahead or just cut her moustache with a fine cuticle scissors immediately before a date.

Electrolysis is virtually permanent hair removal, executed with an electric needle or electric tweezers. It is expensive and time-consuming, but if you have a serious hair problem, especially on your face, it may be worth it. Specialists in this field say that hairs that have been tweezed often have damaged follicles, and in this case the process may have to be repeated several times.

How to find a good electrolysis specialist? Ask a dermatologist. Or get the name from someone who has had successful treatments. Years ago, the procedure used to leave tiny holes in the skin; but now, done by a trained professional with highly specialized equipment the results are really amazing.

The procedure is also used on parts of the body other than the face. Along with the legs and arms, there is the "bikini" wax to remove excess pubic hair for beach lovers.

Not all hair removal is purely aesthetic. Hormonal changes in your body can cause excessive hair growth, so if you are having a serious problem, you may need to see your family doctor and/or an endocrinologist (specialist in hormonal problems).

Chapter 3

HAIR:
HEAD START
ON BEAUTY

aybe it sounds silly, but the best routine is the one that *works*. And what works for you is bound to be different than what works for your best friend.

I started graying when I was twelve. I used to pull out each gray hair as it came in, but soon I realized that if I kept pulling them out, I would have to choose between gray and bald. That's when I gave up the pluck-away project.

I get lots of compliments on my hair, so when Hollywood hair stylist José Eber suggested coloring it, I said no. I keep such a hectic schedule and I'm so lazy, I'd never have time to keep my roots the same color as the rest of my hair! I have had a long blunt cut for several years. Here's how I take care of it. I usually buy whatever shampoo is on sale and change brands every three or four shampoos. In general, some beauty experts say, switching hair products from time to time is a good idea. When I use one product exclusively for a while, my hair seems to stop responding to it.

When I blow-dry my hair, I dry it from underneath, fluffing it up with my fingers and lifting with a brush. The ends dry faster than the roots, and drying from the roots gives more body to hair, so I get more fullness by bending over and drying my hair upside down. I shake my hair as I dry it to get even more body (and a little exercise at the same time).

I'm lucky. My hair is in good condition, which I think comes from care and proper nutrition. Beauty starts on the inside, and poor nutrition or crash dieting can raise havoc with your hair. In fact, a diet of eight hundred calories can cause excessive hair loss.

Because my hair's in such good shape, I only condition it every six months or so, and I like to use a mayonnaise conditioner. You'll find directions for conditioning later in this chapter.

Here are some hair-care ideas I've collected from beauty experts, beauties, and those beautiful people, my readers.

• SHAMPOOING YOUR HAIR •

Most people don't know how to shampoo hair properly. First, dilute your shampoo; most products are too thick. It's easier to wash and rinse with diluted shampoo, and your supply will last longer. (This is an especially good idea if you have young children and teenagers, who really know how to empty a shampoo bottle!)

For starters, get an empty liquid detergent bottle and pour half the shampoo into it. Then fill both the shampoo and liquid detergent bottles with water. Now you've got two bottles of shampoo for the price of one. Or you could use a soft liquid soap dispenser. A dispenser or squirt bottle helps control the application, so that you don't have it pour out in a big glop.

Squirt the shampoo into your hand, rub both hands together, and then apply it to your wet hair. If you pour shampoo directly onto your hair, you'll probably be getting too much, and the glop will be concentrated in just one place so it will not only be difficult to distribute the suds evenly throughout your hair, but will also be even more difficult to rinse properly. Don't forget to make every drop of shampoo count. As the bottle empties, add a little water to mix with any leftover drops of shampoo (or hair rinse).

Shampoo as often as you like. Most people only need to lather up once, especially those who shampoo daily or almost daily. Sudsing just the scalp area is usually enough for those with long hair. Of course, this depends on how long it's been between shampoos, and how dirty your hair is. If you've just finished three games of racketball, or have been out in the sunny yard planting your fall garden, lathering all over is a necessity. You may also need to shampoo more often during the holidays, or if you live in an industrial city. Air pollutants and smoky party rooms tend to make hair dirty faster. Dark, very curly, or chemically colored hair tends to be more porous, absorbing odors and other pollutants quickly.

I have healthy hair, so I can use any kind of shampoo, but researchers suggest that people with dry or damaged hair use a mild, low-Ph shampoo instead of detergent-based shampoo.

• *CONDITIONING YOUR HAIR* •

Condition regularly, especially if you blow-dry or use hot rollers and curling irons often. Permed and colored hair need extra care too. Most of all, protect your hair from summer sun, and always rinse out all salt or chlorinated water after swimming.

If your hair is damaged or dry, condition it weekly. If it's normal, condition every three to six months. It's the dry ends that need the conditioner, not your scalp. Especially with long hair, apply conditioner only to the ends.

Very dry, damaged hair can benefit from an oil pack. Use a polyunsaturated oil (corn, almond, safflower). Warm the oil in a double boiler or, if you warm it in a microwave, use a micro-safe cup. The oil should be warmed to body temperature and should not be hot. Massage it into hair. Put a plastic bag, shower cap, or plastic wrap over your hair, wrap your head in a hot, damp towel for a couple of hours, and hope no unexpected company arrives!

Most treatments need to stay on the hair at least twenty to thirty minutes to be effective. If you've wrapped your hair securely, you can even go to bed that way, allowing the conditioner to work overnight. But be sure the wrap is secure, because some oils stain bed linens. Another way to boost the conditioning treatment is to wrap hair with plastic or put on a shower cap, then sit under a bonnet-style hair dryer for twenty to thirty minutes.

Shampoo with several latherings and rinse. Some people like to rinse with beer after conditioning, followed by a water rinse. If you don't rinse well afterward, the conditioner will leave a dull film on your hair.

Other home-style conditioners are mayonnaise, mashed avocado, egg yolks, and plain yogurt. (Sounds like a salad or a new kind of dip recipe, doesn't it? Just don't add lettuce!) You can use one at a time or mix two or three of the conditioning ingredients for a treatment.

For a protein conditioner that's good for most hair types, mix a tablespoon of sesame (or other light oil) with two egg yolks. Mix well; apply and work into hair; cover with hot, damp towel and leave on for twenty minutes; rinse.

You can also apply coconut or wheat germ oil or petroleum jelly (sparingly) to the ends of your hair to protect them from the summer sun, salt, or chlorine. In general, it's a good idea to use conditioners containing sunscreens if you are very active in summer sports. The sun can change the chemistry of your hair and discolor it—even turn it dry as straw. It's best to cover your hair in the sun, especially if you color your hair. Do yourself a favor and make a habit of picking up your sunglasses and sunhat as you head for the great outdoors.

• COMBS AND BRUSHES •

Never use a brush on wet or damp hair. Brushes are for dry hair only. Current thinking is that those one hundred strokes a night that women have been told to give their hair may actually do more harm than good. This is especially true for dry or damaged hair, which can split and break if brushed too vigorously. Occasional brushing can stimulate your scalp's blood circulation and get your natural oils from the roots to the ends of your hair, and brushing does remove superficial dandruff. But like anything else, moderation is the key.

Some people are in favor of natural bristle brushes; others prefer nylon. Combinations of synthetic and natural bristles are also available. Those who recommend nylon bristles say the bristles of a good hair brush should have widely spaced rounded ends that are held in a flexible rubber pad. This is the kind I use.

If you have a static electricity problem, try using a wide-toothed aluminum comb. For sectioning or combing wet hair, a wide-toothed comb is best. Just start at the bottom and work your way up, unsnarling bad tangles wth your fingers as you go. Avoid pulling and tugging at wet hair.

Cleaning your hair brushes and combs is easy. First, brush hairs out of your comb and comb hairs out of your brush. Here are some tips.

In a mayo jar, mix any of the following in hot water: shampoo, ammonia, ammonia and detergent, baking soda, liquid soap. Shake, soak, shake, scrub, and rinse. Alcohol will cut oil on combs, but test first before using it on synthetic brush bristles. You can toss plastic brushes into the washer, just as long as you don't toss them in with knits or any other fabrics that can get snagged.

• DRYING HAIR •

Hair breaks easily and is very elastic when it's wet. Blot hair with a towel to take out excess water, then wrap your head with the towel to absorb more water. Don't rub harshly.

Hair dryers are great for drying and styling hair, but they must be used carefully. If you're using a hand-held dryer, remember to keep it moving and hold it about six to eight inches away from your hair. Otherwise, you could end up baking a section of your hair with all that hot air. You may need 1,000-watt drying power to do an ordinary drying, but for styling, 750- or 500-watt power is fine.

As I've mentioned, I like to bend over and dry my hair upside down, shaking it for more fullness. You can also section off your hair with a wide-toothed comb and work around your head from one side to the other, drying the front section last. For maximum fullness it's a good idea to work from side to side, pick up your hair layer by layer, and dry it layer by layer, bringing each layer down by twirling it with a styling brush. You can follow the same layering technique on the back of your hair if you bring your hair up and over to one side and hold the dryer over your head as you aim it at the hair. After you bring each layer down, smooth it with a brush.

Here's another way to dry long hair. But first remember that if you are using this method as a straightener for curly hair or just need extra body, apply setting lotion before beginning. Take long clips (not bobby pins or short clips—they'll make your hair kinky). After combing your hair, part it on the left or right. Then wrap your hair toward the part as tightly as you can, using the long metal clips to hold it flat. If you don't make the hair smooth, it will have bumps and kinks after it dries. Wrap your hair around your head as many times as it will go. When dry, remove clips and comb out.

Don't try to sleep on wrapped hair; when you wake up it will be messy.

If you have very long hair, drape a large towel over your shoulders, cape style, to keep your back dry while you comb it.

• STYLING YOUR HAIR •

If you have a naturally curly or permed style, dry your hair without heat; just untangle, style, and shape with your fingers. If hair is very wet, you may want to blow-dry it at the roots for about two minutes; if hair is dry, spritz it with a plant mister. (This is also a good technique for reviving a natural or permed curly style.)

You can use a wide-toothed comb to take out bad tangles.

If you have a layered cut, finger-style it by sections.

If you have a blunt cut, as you work on the hair lift it from the hairline and roots.

Make miniwaves by finger-combing hair and squeezing out any excess moisture against the palm of your hand. It will probably be difficult for you to tell exactly what you are doing on the back of your head, but squeeze and style as best you can. Then let hair air dry naturally.

If you like to set curls reasonably fast, but your hair is too dry or damaged to use hot rollers, try rolling dry hair on perm rods, then get into the shower for a *steam* set—and I mean steam. Don't get your hair wet under the shower head.

Keep in mind that any time you twist your hair before rolling it, it will look fuller when you take out the rollers and comb it.

For an easy new style that will look like a narrow braided hairband, take a section of hair above each ear, twist to form a coil, then draw the coil to the back and top of your head. Hold in place with a comb, barrette, or hairpins. You don't need very long hair for this look.

If you want a temporary frizzy style, either braid your hair while it's wet and let it dry, or twist strands of hair and roll them on perm rods or very small rollers, steam as in the non-hot-roller technique for damaged hair.

To put just a little curl into the ends of long hair, when you go to sleep at night put hair on top of your head in a bun: just bend over and brush all your hair forward, catch it with your hand, then straighten up and twist the hair into a bun. The trick is to dampen the bottom three inches of hair, then wind it tightly around the core of the bun like a giant pincurl. When you brush out hair in the morning, ends will turn under just a little bit. This is what I do when I'm on the road.

Fabric softener sheets are just the right aid for rolling a short, tight, curly style. One sheet makes at least four spongy end papers. These sponge sheets make curlers less torture to sleep on overnight, and in general they work well for anyone who uses rollers—whether their hair is short or long. Remember to dampen both the sponge sheets and your hair before setting.

Store rollers in a clothespin bag and poke roller pins into a plastic mesh pot scrubber ball. Or wash, dry, and store rollers in a mesh fruit bag—you don't even have to take them out of the bag when you wash them!

If you curl your hair with heated rollers, be sure to dry hair first. Hair is so elastic when it is wet that it will shrink tighter around the rollers as it dries and you will end up with curls much tighter than you want—maybe even a frizz. Always wait a minute or so after you remove heated curlers to let curls cool before combing your hair.

Heated curlers dry out the hair, so most hairdressers advise using them only two or three times a week—*not* every day. If you live in an especially humid climate, they will help curl hair that goes limp from the moisture in the air.

If you are not careful electric curling irons can scorch hair. Use them with thermostats and non-stick coatings as a precaution. All you need is a few seconds on each curl. Hairdressers use the irons on a curl until they feel some heat coming through the hair—only a few seconds. Don't use curling irons on bleached or damaged hair.

Did you know you can "iron" your hair straighter as well as make it curly with an electric curling iron? If your perm is too kinky, iron large, fat curls; let hair cool, then comb for a smoother look. Be sure you always use a curling iron on dry hair.

One of the readers of my column suggested that if hair is short and tapered, wrapping it in a nylon net will make it dry flat and neat.

If your hair needs more body, blow-dry until it's slightly damp, then work styling gel through short hair, applying the gel only to the roots if hair is long.

Styling gel is great for setting a few curls here and there to jazz up a style, but if you have to use lots of gel all the time to keep hair in place, the chances are you don't have the right hairstyle. Talk to a stylist to find the look that's attractive and easy to maintain.

Flat beer makes a great setting lotion. Pour it into a mist-spray bottle. Spray on damp hair and set. And don't worry about smelling like a brewery: the odor evaporates.

• *GETTING THE RIGHT STYLE* •

If you can't afford a first-rate hairstylist then the cheapest way to get expert consultation is to go to a school that trains hair stylists. A student may work on your hair, but the work will be supervised by an instructor who is likely to be up on the newest techniques and styles.

One way to find a new stylist is to look for someone who has hair similar to yours or a hairstyle that you like. When you go to the hairdresser, take along a picture of the style you want, but don't expect to end up looking exactly like the model in the picture—unless, that is, you two are identical twins. Hair texture and type influence the look of a cut as much as the stylist's skill.

The fall is a good time to have hair styled, so that sun-damaged hair gets cut off as hair is being shaped. And it's usually better to get your hair cut before you leave on vacation so it's done by a hairdresser who knows your hair and you don't have to take a chance with a stranger.

Getting hair styled can be an adventure. It certainly was when I had mine done by the famous Hollywood stylist José Eber. He really plays with hair—moving it around, pushing and pulling it from top to bottom, lifting, fluffing. And when he had finished "arranging" my hair, he stepped back as we both looked at it in the mirror from all angles to see if we liked the concept. He even tried me with bangs—all before he did any actual cutting. He took great pains to make sure the hairstyle flattered the shape of my face and suited my height and weight. He also observed the texture and body of my hair, and the direction in which each hair section grows, as well as how the style would highlight the color of my hair.

He asked me about my life-style to find out how much time I have to fool around with my hair each day. (Not much!) He wanted to know how often I shampoo, if I used a blow dryer, curling irons, hot rollers, and if I have time to go to the beauty shop regularly. When he finally did cut and style my hair, we both knew we'd like the results: he cut several inches off and layered it all around in long layers.

When you are choosing a new hairstyle, think about your life-style.

Do you go to the beauty salon every week?

Do you have such a busy schedule that all you can do is shampoo and air dry?

Are you comfortable using blow dryers, hot rollers, and curling irons?

How often do you need to shampoo and condition your oily or dry hair?

Do you like to fuss with your hair, or just comb it in the morning and forget it?

If you and your hairdresser base selection of a hairstyle on life-style as well as looks, you'll probably be as thrilled with your new hairdo as I was with mine.

It's a relief to many women to know that age no longer decides the length of your hair. The length is selected according to your face, neck length, body structure, and type of hair. Softer styles are usually more flattering to older women, but the choice is an individual one.

Generally, short hair needs a maintenance cut every three to four weeks. And even if you are letting your hair grow, you should get a trim every four to six weeks just to avoid split ends. Most short hair styles are layered cuts.

Although some people with medium-length hair will find they need a perm to maintain it, in general this length hair is the most practical.

• *HAIR COLORING* •

If your life-style is a busy one, as is mine, you should think carefully about coloring your hair. You could settle instead for having hair lightened via streaking, highlighting, or hair painting. This way you wouldn't have to worry about dark roots showing every few weeks. Or you could try a natural hair coloring that fades slightly with each shampoo.

If you have gray hair and use a color rinse, but want a light streak at the temples, here's how to do it yourself. Wind up one or more strands at the front—the ones you want to be light—and wrap them in aluminum foil. Then, as directed, apply your color. After your hair has processed, unwrap the foil-covered strands, and— *violà*—you'll have a light streak.

To prevent hair dye from staining skin, smooth petroleum jelly on your forehead and around the sides of your face *before* you color.

Henna is considered a "natural" hair-coloring product because it's made from a plant root and stems. It not only can improve your hair's body and sheen, but it also accents its color. You can buy henna in shades of black, brown and red, and neutral. The neutral (I use it on my gray hair) adds sheen without changing hair color.

But henna isn't for everyone. Some henna preparations can interfere with the chemical processes of perms, so be sure to tell your hairdresser if you are using any henna products before you get a perm. If you are giving yourself a home permanent, check with the instructions on the label to see if henna can affect the perm's chemicals.

If you don't use henna as directed, you can damage your hair. Blondes and others with light-tinted hair should be especially careful about following directions when using henna. It can, for example, turn gray hair orange. And *don't* mix henna with other hair-coloring products—you may end up with a color that you cry over.

Coloring your hair can give you a psychological lift, but remember that colored hair needs special care. Always cover colored hair when you're in the sun, and that includes when you're playing tennis, riding in a convertible, or relaxing on the beach. If you're not careful, brown hair tones can turn red in the sun, whereas blond tones can become orange or green. The emergency treatment for sun-discolored dyed hair is to use a temporary color rinse that washes out with the next shampoo. Such temporary rinses won't penetrate or change the hair shaft structure, so they won't damage hair.

Apply a conditioner to colored hair *every* time you shampoo. If you apply coloring at home, avoid using a very hot dryer imediately afterward. Set the temperature at low.

Many colorists suggest choosing a hair color no more than four or five shades lighter or darker than your original color for the most "natural" look. You can brighten up light brown hair with copper or caramel shades; mahogany, chestnut, and auburn will brighten drab and dull brunette hair.

And remember, if you change your hair color, you also may need to change the rest of you. Your eye makeup, for example. Take everything into account.

Here are some other general hair-coloring rules:

• Stark black should be avoided because it looks artificial and accents lines on the face.

• If you choose a subtle tone, a shade or so lighter than your natural tone, touch-ups won't be needed as often.

• As you get older, lighter tones are more flattering to the skin.

• Because perm solutions alter color, get perms before getting color.

• Condition hair well before and after a permanent hair coloring, and always wait at least four weeks between color applications. Putting one dye on top of another can have disastrous results, creating color never meant for hair. I've seen women come into the beauty salon with honest-to-gosh green hair after home-coloring mistakes.

Here are some definitions of the different types of coloring:

• *Streaking, Highlighting, Hair Painting:* small amounts of hair are bleached and toned, often imitating nature's way of sun streaking at the crown or framing your face with color that is lighter than the rest of your hair.

• *Color Rinse:* products that lightly coat the hair shaft with color until shampooed out.

• *Semipermanent Tints:* these actually penetate the hair shaft, but only stay on the hair for about a month.

• *Permanent Tint:* these penetrate deep into the hair shaft and need time to grow out.

• *Sun Coloring or Bleaching:* exercise caution with this approach. In fact, if you have poorly conditioned hair, I suggest that you avoid it altogether. Some people dab lemon juice or a mixture of lemon juice and a few drops of peroxide and almond or coconut oil on their hair before outdoor activities such as swimming or gardening and then let the sun do the bleaching/streaking color process. Follow up with a shampoo and conditioning treatment.

When you are selecting a hair color, remember that the swatches of hair samples you see at the salon or color shown on packages of home-coloring products show the color when applied to white hair or hair that has been stripped of its color. Read the packages of home-coloring products carefully to find out how the color looks when applied to *your* hair shade. At the salon, you'll have to trust your hairdresser, but make sure you've picked someone you *can* trust: not all hairdressers are proficient in coloring.

• *TO PERM OR NOT TO PERM* •

Famous hairdressers agree that a good haircut can give you a style that doesn't need a perm, but even these experts will admit that there are many women (and men) who need a body perm for the look they want. Once you and your hairdresser hit upon the right perm solution for your hair, keep records of it so that you get the same result every time. If you perm at home, or change hairdressers, keep your own records.

If you perm your hair yourself, trim off the old perm before getting a new one to avoid damaging your hair. Also, the days of letting a perm "grow out" are over. You'll need regular trims to keep hair healthy and in shape. With regular trimming a perm lasts about six months.

Always read instructions carefully when you give yourself a home perm. Most will tell you to section off a strand almost as wide as the rod and about one-half inch deep. Then saturate your hair with waving lotion or water, as directed. End papers should be folded over the bottom of hair strands, and curls should be wound firmly.

Here are two good home-perm hints from my readers. Cream your face before starting the perm to prevent waving solution from burning your skin if it runs down your face. And roll the curl just above your forehead forward instead of back (like the rest) to avoid forming a ridge.

Check with your hairdresser; many hairdressers advise not washing hair for three to four days after a perm to allow it to stabilize. Washing hair too soon after a perm can cause it to relax and lose curl.

• *SPECIAL PROBLEMS, SPECIAL SOLUTIONS* •

If you have days when you really do feel, "I can't do a thing with my hair," take heart. Hairdressers have solutions to most problems and many of them you can learn to do yourself.

Here are some common complaints and solutions:

• *Oily Hair:* shampoo more often. Try leaving lather on for about two to five minutes before rinsing. Use warm, never hot, water; hot water stimulates oil glands. Put conditioners on ends only. Wear a hairstyle that requires minimum effort. Wash combs and brushes clean every week (actually, this is good advice whatever your hair type).

• *Dry Hair:* don't overprocess or overdry hair. Do use conditioners or special setting lotions that give a sheen. Use a wide-tooth comb. Curling irons will add shine by closing the cuticle of your hair. Keep your hair short with frequent trims.

• *Thin or Fine Hair:* shampoo often. Use setting gels, good perms, hair coloring. Set with small curlers to get more body.

• *Coarse Hair:* have a layered cut. Avoid harsh perms or coloring products. Condition regularly. Add shine with hot curlers and curling irons.

• *Dull Hair:* avoid sun and harsh treatment with combs and brushes. Use a deep conditioner often, and look for sprays and products that say they add shine. Hot rollers and curling irons help with shine, too.

• *Limp Hair:* shampoo often. Dilute conditioners by half and use them only on the ends of your hair. Styling gels add body, as does a perm.

• *Straight Hair:* try a layered cut or treat yourself to a good perm. Use setting lotion with hot rollers or curling iron.

• *Frizzy, Too Curly Hair:* use styling gels. Comb with a pick to avoid pulling through tangles. Get a good cut, and use creamy shampoos and conditioners. Use conditioners with extra protein. Try this special protein moisturizer: mix two tablespoons each of mayonnaise and safflower oil with two egg yolks. Comb through hair; leave on for half an hour; shampoo out.

• *Static Electricity in Hair:* use an aluminum, wide-tooth comb. Apply water-base instant conditioner after shampoo.

• *Growing Short Hair Out:* this will really test your patience! It takes about four months for a short, layered hairstyle to grow into a long style. If you are growing your layered style to a single length, you'll need to have the bottom layers trimmed as they grow. Get a soft perm and use barrettes, combs, and headbands for control during the transition period.

Here's a trick to prevent hair that gets limp as it's growing out:

condition the ends *before* you shampoo. And for any part of your hair that sticks out during the growing process, use setting gel. Apply the gel, then comb neckline hairs back so they won't hang beneath your ears.

Mostly, be patient; in four months, your hair should grow about two inches, but it will probably take six or more months to get you from short to longer hair.

· *KITCHEN RINSES AND REMEDIES* ·

• *Dandruff:* try this old folk/kitchen remedy. Make a "tea" by adding about one tablespoon of chives to one-half cup water. Strain, cool, use as a scalp rinse.

• *Sheen:* try an old favorite, fresh lemon juice.

• *Dark-Hair Rinses:* simmer one teaspoon allspice, one teaspoon crushed cinnamon stick, and one-half teaspoon cloves in one cup water. Strain, cool, and then rinse.

Also, add about one-fourth cup rosemary to one quart of boiling water, steep until mixture has strong aroma and color; cool; strain; use as final rinse.

• *Light-Hair Rinse:* add about one-fourth cup chamomile tea or flowers to one quart of water; follow instructions for rosemary rinse.

• *Oily-Hair Rinse:* after shampoo, rinse with an acidic liquid, such as one-fourth cup lemon juice or one-fourth cup cider vinegar to one quarter water.

• *Rosemary Conditioner:* steep two tablespoons of rosemary in one cup cold milk for three hours; strain out rosemary; add one whole egg and one tablespoon honey. Rub into hair; cover with plastic wrap or shower cap and leave on for one hour; shampoo.

Mashed avocado can be added to the rosemary-and-milk mixture. Follow the same application and removal instructions.

• *Oil Treatments from the Kitchen:* combine olive, almond, peanut, safflower, walnut, or wheat germ oils with any of the following spices: lavender, rosemary, oregano, nutmeg, sage, nettle, clove, comfrey, burdock. Warm the oil, simmer with herb of your choice for about thirty minutes; strain; cool only slightly—it should be warm when you put it on hair and scalp. Wrap your head in a hot towel and plastic wrap or shower cap for thirty minutes; shampoo twice.

And don't forget about my favorite oil treatment: mayonnaise. But use it only on the ends of your hair.

• OTHER TIPS AND QUICK FIXES •

• *Yellow Tinge:* a yellow tinge on gray or white hair can be caused by pollution, nicotine, perspiration, or other chemicals in the body or the environment. Try shampooing more often to see if pollutants are the problem.

• *Green Tint in Blond Hair:* the copper—not the chlorine—in pools and freshwater lakes can give blond a greenish tint. Wear a swimcap and, immediately afterward, rinse hair with club soda. The carbon dioxide in the soda lifts out the copper.

• *Limp Hair:* is hair limp even a day after you've shampooed? Stop using fabric softeners on your towels. One of my readers discovered that the residue of the fabric softener in towels and bed linens also softened her hair.

If yours is the kind of hairstyle that really goes limp in damp weather, don't squash it down with a hat to protect it. Try using a light silky scarf, tied loosely. Combs and barrettes, lifting hair into an asymmetrical style, are helpful, too.

Here's another tip: If your curly or permed hair looks limp, mist your hair with your plant mister, then fluff up your curls with your fingers. *Don't brush!*

• *Make Rollers:* caught without enough rollers for your hair? Or need disposable rollers when you are traveling? Try using strips of cloth or tissue paper, or facial tissue or aluminum foil. Tie the cloth to the end of a hair strand; roll the curl to the scalp; tie, and let dry. Roll on paper, facial tissue, or foil in similar fashion.

• *Quick Fix:* here's a quick fix for droopy hair that will last at least for one evening out. Fluff up or tease hair; then bend over and shake hair; spray hair from underneath; shake hair with your fingers; hold your head up again, and comb.

Remember that hair sprays help fine hair keep its shape in bad weather, but you should always brush lacquer out of your hair when you get back indoors. According to some experts, hair sprays dry your hair.

• *Dress-up Ideas:* any length hair is glamorized by a hat, veil, or other accessories. For example, wear a tiara, headband, flower, barrette, decorated comb, or ribbon. You can also use a fabric belt from a dress, a gold cord, or a pearl or beaded necklace twisted into your hair.

Don't be afraid to jazz up your everyday hairstyle for evening by putting up just a section of hair, braiding or twisting a section, or trying an off-center ponytail.

• *Wig-wearing Tip:* if you are buying a wig after a dramatic hair loss (due to illness or chemotherapy), wait as long as you can *before* you buy; the more hair you have when you buy the wig, the looser it's going to be if you lose more hair. Buy the best you can afford, so you will feel good about wearing the wig. And this is *not* the time to take on a radically new color or style—you'll just call attention to the very problem you're trying to conceal.

• *SPLIT ENDS* •

If you have long hair, split ends could be the bane of your existence. Braid your hair with simple three-strand braids, making one or as many braids as you need to match the volume of your hair. Have a friend hold the end of the braid with one hand, while gently rubbing the other hand upward on the braid from the tip toward the scalp. This action will cause the split ends to pop out of the braids. Carefully trim the bristly-looking split end tips, being careful *not to cut* into the braid. Some women simply twist sections of hair, instead of braiding them.

There is evidence that we are genetically programmed to have a certain hair length and then when our hair reaches this length, the ends begin to split. If you are troubled by split ends at a certain hair length, you may be programmed by Mom Nature to wear a shorter hair style—one compatible with the natural maximum length your hair grows without split ends.

The best way to avoid split ends is by getting the ends of your hair trimmed monthly, or every six to eight weeks, depending on how fast your hair grows. Even long hair needs to have a fourth of an inch cut off about every two months to keep it looking good.

• *HAIR GROWTH AND LOSS* •

Most hair grows about one-half to three-quarters of an inch each month. And did you know that hair, like autumn leaves, falls in a cyclical pattern? You'll lose the most hair in November and the least in May.

When a single hair has been growing on your head for about three years, it simply stops growing, rests for about three months, and then falls out. A new hair grows in the same hair follicle.

If you think you are losing more hair than you normally do, some cosmetologists suggest that you count the hairs that have collected on your comb. If there are more than one hundred, you ought to consult a competent hair-care expert. Chemicals in perms and coloring products could be causing excessive hair loss.

You can tell if hair is falling out or just breaking off by checking the ends of the hair. If a white bulb is at the end, the hair has fallen out. If there is no white end, and you can feel stubble on your scalp, hairs are breaking off. In either case, you should check any new hair products you are using and, if the loss continues, see your doctor. Certain diseases, illnesses, nutritional problems, and medications can affect your hair's health.

Chapter 4

RX FOR EYES

You only have to look at your eyes to see what's going on with the rest of you. When you're sick, tired, allergic, or unhappy, they show it; and just as dramatically they tell the world when they're bright and sparkling that you're on the top of the world and life's A-OK.

If your eyes itch, hurt, are red, puffy, runny, or show any out-of-the-ordinary symptoms, and if the usual common remedies—pads or drops—don't help, see your ophthalmologist or optometrist.

An optometrist is a doctor trained to prescribe glasses and recognize eye diseases. When an optometrist spots a problem that needs special treatment, he or she refers you to an ophthalmologist. An ophthalmologist is a physician who specializes in diseases of and surgery on the eyes.

Did you know that glaucoma can begin its damaging course when you are as young as thirty? Seeing a doctor about eye problems—and on a regular basis if you wear glasses or contact lenses —is one of the better investments in your vision's future.

· PUFFY PROBLEM ·

If you read beauty columns in magazines and newspapers, you're sure to have heard the question, "What do I do about puffy eyes?"

If this is one of those problems you face every morning, raise the head of your bed (if you have a waterbed, forget it). Why? When you lie down flat, your body is like a salt table, and the fluid seeks the lowest level. With your head up as you sleep, you will prevent the fluid from collecting in your head and causing under-eye puffiness. You don't have to make it a dramatic lift—all you need is a few inches. A few books or small pieces of wood under the legs of the bed headboard will suffice. You can also try sleeping on two pillows to raise your head. Since my husband and I have a waterbed, this is what I do. However, sleeping on two pillows may give you a neckache, so it's best if you can raise the whole bed.

How to tell what's causing puffy eyes—fluid accumulation, an allergy, irritant, or health problem? Observe what happens to the puffs after you've been awake and upright for a few hours. If they vanish, it's fluid accumulating. In addition to raising your head at night, decreasing your salt intake would help. But if puffy under-eyes stay puffed all day, the chances are you're having an allergic reaction, or some other problem. See your doctor just to make sure it's nothing serious.

· UNDER-EYE BAGS ·

Under-eye bags are another common beauty problem, just as disfiguring as under-eye puffiness. And what's worse is that they won't go away, because they're filled with fatty deposits, not fluid. If getting more sleep, avoiding alcohol, and in general adopting a healthier life-style doesn't deflate your under-eye bags, your only alternative may be plastic surgery—specifically, an operation called a blepharoplasty. Just pronouncing it is enough to give you bags under the eyes!

For information about plastic surgery, write to: American Society of Plastic and Reconstructive Surgery, 233 N. Michigan Avenue, Chicago, IL 60601. (See Chapter 13.)

Some eye problems will vanish with just a little help from you. But, when it comes to problems that persist, listen to your friend Heloise. See a doctor. Your eyesight is too precious to endanger through neglect.

• HOME REMEDIES •

Beauty treatments for your eyes can be whipped up at home with aids from your pantry shelf or fridge.

Milk Bath

Soak cotton balls or makeup pads in cool skim (not whole) milk. Place on closed eyes for five to ten minutes; remove for two minutes; repeat. This is also soothing if your eyes are irritated or swollen after a good cry. (Come to think of it, who ever has a "good" cry?)

Eye Bags

Lots of women claim that there's nothing like witch hazel pads or tea bags (chamomile tea's my favorite) to ease under-eye puffiness. Place pads or bags over closed eyes while you rest. Both have astringent qualities. If you stash the witch hazel, brewed tea, or used teabags in the fridge, they'll be especially soothing.

Eye Resting

To give your eyes a beautifying break during the day, lie down, feet up, and place damp, cool tea bags on them. The tea's tannic acid acts as an astringent to soothe your eyes and reduce swelling. With or without tea bags, a rest period really helps on a busy day, especially if you have a busy evening ahead of you.

Veggie Treats

Did you know that potato slices (chilled are best) placed directly on the lids help reduce under-eye puffiness?

Cucumber Slices

Cucumber slices feel even cooler when they're chilled. Placed over eyes, they're refreshing, and they ease itchiness.

• *EYE SAFETY AND HEALTH* •

Don't share. That's the best eye-care advice you'll ever get. *Do not* use anyone else's eye makeup. Don't even try on another person's eyeglasses. Why? Diseases and infections can spread when you share. Some cosmetologists even recommend that when you remove eye makeup, you use a fresh cotton ball for each eye to avoid transferring germs from one eye to the other. For the same reason, cotton swabs make good makeup applicators. Be sure to throw them away after each use.

Drops Help

Blood vessels swell when eyes get irritated and sometimes that means red eyes. Just about any over-the-counter eyedrop will relieve the redness. Commercial eyedrops contain a decongestant that constricts blood vessels to eliminate the redness, but regular use of decongestants can cause a "rebound effect" and the blood vessels will enlarge again in less and less time. Use decongestant eyedrops *sparingly*.

• *MAKEUP REMOVAL* •

Remove eye makeup by patting cleanser on closed eyelids and lashes; wipe lightly with a damp natural sponge or soft cotton. Some cosmetologists say that because of its wood content, tissue is too harsh for the delicate skin around your eyes.

Nonirritating Aids

The two safest nonirritating eye makeup (or other makeup) removers that just about anyone can use—even those whose skin is acne-prone—are mineral oil and petroleum jelly. Splash well with water after removing makeup.

One prominent dermatologist says that because it's so inexpensive, the value of mineral oil as a skin sealer or makeup remover is often underrated. Many women find baby oil a great eye makeup remover. It's also less expensive than products made specifically for removing eye makeup.

• *KNOWN IRRITANTS* •

The ingredients in nail polish can irritate your eyes, so always wait until your polish is dry before making up your eyes. Otherwise you could mess up your nails and eyes at the same time, and who needs that?

• *"SOMETHING IN YOUR EYE?"* •

If you get an eyelash or speck in your eye, try rinsing it out with an eyewash solution. If you are very careful, you may be able to catch the lash or speck with a moistened cotton swab. (Getting a helper is a good idea.) If it's on the upper lid, sometimes you can get it out by gently pulling the upper lid over the lower, then blowing your nose. (Believe it or not!) This is not a good idea, however, if you're wearing mascara, because the mascara may irritate your inner lid as much as the dirt.

To rinse eyes irritated by dust, you can use eyewash in a little cup (fill it and place over your eye), or the kind of drops sold for contact lens wearers.

Be sure to check all eyewash or eyedrops before you use them. Liquid should be clear when you hold it to the light—no floating particles or lint. Always wash eyecups, and don't use any dropper or bottle that isn't absolutely clean. Keep containers closed tightly to keep bacteria out. Do not keep eyedrops or wash beyond a year; actually, just to be on the safe side, three months is long enough.

• *DRY EYES* •

Eyes that are chronically red and feel as if there is always something in them can be the result of hormone changes in your body that slow down tear production. This often happens to women over forty. If it happens to you, see your doctor. You may be able to get relief from prescription "artificial tears." Dry eyes can also indicate other health problems, such as rheumatoid arthritis, so don't try to treat this problem yourself.

• STY IN THE EYE •

A sty is an infected oil-secreting gland in the eyelid. Try warm water compresses, with or without an eye ointment that's been recommended by your doctor. They'll help relieve some of the discomfort. For any large or especially painful sties, see your doctor.

• PINKEYE •

Conjunctivitis is a painless infection of the eye's membranes that makes your eyes look red. It may be complicated by a discharge from the eye. See your doctor.

I seem to be prone to conjunctivitis. One night I woke up with my eyes almost closed shut because of the discharge. I took off all of my makeup, rinsed my eyes well, put eye drops in them, and then went to sleep. Four hours later, when I woke up, my eyes looked like the night of the living dead. They were so red and runny that I thought I was having an allergic reaction to something. So, I put in drops and went about my business and a few hours later my eyes were still just as red and runny as before.

I went to see my eye doctor. He told me I had conjunctivitis.

Swell, I thought, I have a TV show to do in two days in Washington, and I'm going to look like I've been up for days. The doctor gave me some eyedrops and said that my eyes should clear in about four or five days.

I was having new glasses made at the time, so I called the store and asked if they could please make just the top part of my glasses slightly pink. Yes, I was going to see the world, or at least Washington, through rose-colored glasses, but the world wasn't going to see my "pink eyes."

Now I always carry my drops on the road, and if conjunctivitis does strike, and I don't have my rose-colored glasses with me, I just pop into a dime store and pick up a pair of tinted glasses.

• *TAKE CARE* •

If you are treating your face to a masque, acne peel, a scrubbing with beauty grains or similar treatment, pretend you are wearing large sunglasses. Do not let any rough or harsh products get closer to your eyes than the outline of your pretend sunspecs.

• *IF YOU WEAR GLASSES* •

Cleaning Lenses

A drop of vinegar on a tissue cleans glass lenses, but *don't* use it on plastic lenses.

Warm water *without* any soap (which leaves a film) will clean glass *or* plastic lenses. Dry with a lint-free cloth.

Beware Scratches

Looking through scratched eyeglass lenses can make your eyes tired and can cause blurred vision. Here's a home remedy for those fine scratches that result from tossing your glasses in your purse or resting them on the lenses instead of keeping them in their case. Make a creamy paste of talcum powder and water in a small dish. Then tissue the paste gently on both sides of the lenses and wipe off. The talc is just abrasive enough to polish out tiny scratches, without causing new ones.

Choosing Frames

There are all sorts of rules for choosing flattering frames for prescription glasses or sunglasses. Most rules are so complicated that it seems simpler to pick up any old frame so long as it doesn't slide off your nose. Here's an easy guide to frame and color selection.

Draw an imaginary horizontal line through the center of the glasses where the lenses will go and where you would expect to see your eyes centered. If the bridge of the glasses is far above the imaginary line, you have high-bridge frames; if the bridge of the glasses is not far from the line, you have low-bridge frames. To make a short nose look longer, buy high-bridge frames; to make a long nose look shorter, buy a low-bridge frame.

COLOR-SCHEMING CUES   When you choose the color of your frames, remember that:

A dark-toned bridge will make a wide nose look narrower.

Frames with light tones in the center that darken out at the edges will make close-set eyes appear wider.

Decorations on the outer edges of lenses, such as gold initials, will draw the eye of the beholder outward too.

For frames that complement your hair and skin tones, here's another handy guide: pale-skinned blondes generally look best in rose, blue, green, and tortoise frames. Olive-skinned brunettes look best in browns, plum, rose, and blue. Tawny-skinned redheads look great in tortoise, green, coral, brown, or amber. And black skin and hair is best heightened by rose and purple or amber.

If you change your hair color often, perhaps metal frames would be the best for you—they're the most basic.

Don't forget that when your hair changes color naturally, you'll need to change the color of your frames too. I used to have dark hair and wear tortoise frames all the time, but my friendly optical specialist suggested that with my light silver hair, I should wear wire frames.

Protecting Frames

One of my readers solved the problem of staining her glasses frames with hair dye by wrapping the ear pieces of her glasses with aluminum foil when her hair is being colored. It keeps the dye off.

Another reader, who found her hair spray was making white spots on her dark-framed glasses, washed them with warm water and soap, dried them thoroughly, and then coated the frames with a thin film of petroleum jelly and polished them. (Petroleum jelly is fast becoming almost as indispensable in my home as vinegar!) Make sure not to get petroleum jelly on the lenses though! You won't have to use this tip if you take your glasses off when you spray your hair.

Lost and Found

Here's a good hint for you poor myopic souls who can't find your glasses without your glasses: attach an eyeglass case near the place where you normally take off your glasses—taped to the nightstand beside your bed or tacked to the wall near the sink where you usually wash your face. This way, the glasses can easily be put into the case and found when you need them. One of my readers lamented that once he stepped on his glasses while he was looking for them because he had knocked them off the nightstand in his sleep and couldn't find them in the morning. Eyeglasses are really expensive these days, well worth a nail in the wall or tape on furniture.

In the Sun

Did you know that wearing clear prescription eyeglasses out in the sun can make dark circles under your eyes darker? The clear glass allows sun rays to beat down on your under-eye area, where the skin is very thin. If you have dark circles, they'll just get darker.

Apply a sunscreen to this delicate skin, but take care not to get it into your eyes.

Better yet, if you are out in the sun a lot, get your prescription made up with dark sun lenses to filter out the sun's rays.

About Lenses

Some optic researchers say that photosensitive or gradient lenses —prescription lenses that darken in sunlight—are worse than no protection at all from the sun because they allow the eyes to relax, while letting in ultraviolet light. Other experts suggest that photosensitive and gradient lenses might be okay for wearing around town, but warn that they are not dark enough to wear near water at the beach where sun is reflected by sand and surf and is more damaging.

Most doctors recommend medium to dark gray lenses, which protect your eyes from the sun without distorting colors. Brown is also considered good, even if it changes colors somewhat. Pink and blue lenses are great fun, but they distort colors and don't screen out the sun's ultraviolet light. Pink lenses might be helpful, however, in reducing the glare of fluorescent lights in an office.

Shopping Savvy

When buying a new pair of nonprescription sunglasses, hold them at arms length, look at any straight line in the store—a shelf, the doorway, a window frame—and see if the line looks wavy or uneven. If it does, your eyes will probably tire when wearing the glasses. Also check carefully to make sure both lenses are the same shade and that they have no scratches or air bubbles that might irritate your eyes.

Sticker of Quality

Some manufacturers put stickers on their glasses to indicate they have met the sunglasses industry's voluntary standards for eliminating ultraviolet light. This standard requires that the sunglasses transmit a percentage of ultraviolet light no higher than that of visible light. This means that if the sunglasses eliminate 25 percent of the visible light, they must also absorb at least 25 percent of the ultraviolet light.

The stickers, which are not required, will indicate the percentage of ultraviolet light eliminated by the glasses. What are the standards? They vary. Quality glasses eliminate 99 percent of the ultraviolet light, but there are many inferior brands that don't come close. Drugstore sunglasses, for example, absorb about 75 percent of the ultraviolet light.

Polarizing glasses eliminate glare from water, but don't always absorb ultraviolet light, so look for the rating sticker.

In general, lenses with mirrored surfaces absorb and reflect ultraviolet light better than regular sunglasses, and glass lenses absorb better than plastic.

• CONTACT LENSES •

Lots of people seem to lose their contact lenses when they're cleaning them. Well, listen to this hint from one of my readers: use a small spice or herb jar with a perforated plastic lid to wash lenses, drain the water through the perforations, and rinse in the same manner—all with no risk of losing the lenses down the drain. Another tip: put a towel or washcloth in the sink before you begin.

Sometimes, despite the best precautions, those sneaky contacts go. Here's what one of my readers did: she took a long-handled screwdriver, wrapped absorbent cotton around it, and stuck it as far down the drain as it would go. The lens stuck to the cotton and —bravo!—up it came.

And think about this: if you cover the end of your vacuum cleaner nozzle with nylon net or old pantyhose, you may actually be able to *vacuum* up a lost contact. Try shining a flashlight around the area where you think you've dropped the lens—the light reflecting off it will tell you where it's fallen.

The best way to avoid all of this is to take those extra few minutes as you're putting in or removing your contact lenses. Don't rush. Replacing lost or damaged lenses is time-consuming and costly.

Applying Makeup

Most contact wearers tell me they insert lenses before putting on makeup. Do remember to *always* wash your hands well before inserting contacts.

Look for eye makeup with a label saying, "Ophthalmologist-tested—safe with contact lenses."

Beware of iridescent eye shadows—they're made with ground-up mother-of-pearl and can cause problems if the material flecks into your eyes.

Creamy stick shadows work well with contact lenses; there's no irritating powder to fleck into your eye.

Don't line the inside of your eyelids with pencil—the wax can block glands and get onto your lenses. Stick to the outside of your lids. (For more makeup hints, go to Chapter 8.)

• EYEBROWS •

Eyebrow Tweezing

Fighting the battle of the brows is enough to drive almost any woman to tears, especially if she's inherited the tendency to grow one brow—straight across over both eyes. And it's kind of hard to see which hairs to pluck when you're weeping from the plucking pain of it all!

Believe me, painless or almost painless plucking *is* possible. Here's how.

Don't just attack your face with tweezers! If skin is very sensitive, *prepare* it first: rub the area with the formula they sell to numb a teething baby's gums, or numb skin by rubbing an ice cube over the area. You can also relax the skin around the brows *before* you start by applying a washcloth or cotton balls that have been dipped in warm water. Heat helps open the pores.

After your skin has softened, get out your brow brush or an extra toothbrush (not the one you use on your teeth, of course), and if you're planning on tweezing the area above the brow, brush brows down; if it's below the brow that you're concerned about, brush brows up. Be sure to move back and forth, eye to eye, so that you don't end up with lopsided brows.

The general rule for tweezing: the highest point of the brow should be in the arch just above the point where your iris (colored area) meets the white, on the outer corner.

Taming Brows

When you are finished, wipe the brow area with an astringent, and brush brows into shape. A little hair spray on your brush helps tame unruly brows. And for those rebellious brows that sneak into a droop as the day goes on, brush them into an arch and hold them in place by lightly applying water or smudge-proof mascara with the mascara applicator. This will help them stay put all day. I got this tip from a friend who has black brows and lashes and uses dark brown or brownish-black mascara on lashes and brows. She doesn't use eyebrow pencil.

Soap is also an eyebrow tamer. Rub a clean mascara brush on a wet bar of soap and brush brows into place with the slightly soaped brush.

Have you ever noticed that a few eyebrow hairs seem to pop up out of nowhere *after* you're all made up? (What few? I could make a hairpiece from all the hairs I've plucked from my eyebrows.) Well, if it really is only a few, I go ahead and pluck them—as long as it's not going to mess up my eye shadow or make my eyebrow line red.

Brow Shape-up

Your eyebrows frame your face, so shaping them is important. Let's face it, one thick long brow makes you look as if you're angry! Brows need to be separated. Even the current full look is not shaggy. Beauty experts recommend natural shapes. That almost-no-brows-at-all look is dated, and you know what happens when you wear a look from the past—you look like you belong there! Most beauty consultants agree that your brows should arch at the corners to give you an uplifted look. Droopy brows make you look sad and tired. Round, full faces need brows that make a definite peak to add angular lines to that roundness.

Eyebrow pencil helps to fill in and create the shape you need for your face. (For more how-tos, see Chapter 8.)

Grow-outs

It takes about three months for eyebrows to grow out. If you want to grow your brows without looking like a plucked chicken, try facial bleach on the hairs you would normally pluck. But be careful to keep the bleach away from your eyes *and* the delicate skin around your eyes.

Bleaching Brows

Facial bleach is also used to lighten brows to better match hair color. Mix the bleach as directed on the package; apply to brows for two minutes *only*. Then remove bleach with a tissue, and carefully wash the area with mild soap and water. Remove any residue of bleach by dabbing the area with a cotton ball soaked in alcohol, again being careful not to let the alcohol in your eyes.

The hairs will get lighter than they appear immediately after the bleaching session, so don't overdo it. Otherwise, you'll end up with brows so light-colored that nobody will be able to see them!

Chapter 5

TEETH: SAFEGUARD YOUR SMILE

once met someone who never brushed her lower teeth because she said that they didn't show when she smiled. Well, they sure did. And I can tell you, it wasn't a pretty picture.

Did you know that keeping your teeth actually helps you live longer? That's because people who can chew their food tend to eat more nutritious foods. Of course, people who take care of their teeth are likely to take care of the rest of their bodies, too. So proper tooth care is more than cosmetic—it's healthy.

Just as teeth help you maintain good nutrition, good nutrition helps you maintain good teeth. Some new studies at the University of Rochester School of Medicine and Dentistry in New York by William H. Bowen, Ph.D., show that the amount of sugar you eat is not as important as *when* and *what* kind of sugary food you eat. Dentists and dental researchers say, if you must eat sugary foods, eat them with meals; don't munch on them constantly throughout the day—that provides the perfect environment for decay-producing bacteria to settle in, thrive, and go about their nasty work.

Mouth bacteria start to work immediately after you eat sweets. If you don't neutralize the decay-causing acids the bacteria produce, these acids work on your teeth for twenty minutes, at which point saliva neutralizes them. If you don't give saliva a chance to come to the rescue—if you eat sweets nonstop—you'll get cavities. Every time you pop a piece of candy into your mouth the process starts all over again. If you ate a sugary food every twenty minutes you could keep your teeth in a decay-causing situation all day long. A little extreme, maybe, but you get my point.

• *FIGHTING TOOTH DECAY* •

Eat sweets with meals and brush and floss afterward. Avoid sugary snacks at bedtime; always brush and floss before you go to sleep—saliva flows less at night, and decay-causing bacteria will have a field day if left in your mouth all night long.

Eat cheese after sweets. Recent studies show that cheddar and other aged cheeses protect tooth enamel. So, have dessert European-style; and follow sweets with a morsel of cheese.

Avoid gooey sweets that stick to your teeth, such as caramels, and even dried fruits, honey, peanut butter and jelly. If you must indulge, brush and floss afterward.

When you can't brush, eat a high-fiber food at the end of a meal, such as an apple, celery, cucumber, lettuce. Fibrous foods increase saliva flow, thereby neutralizing the acids that cause decay. Other foods that increase saliva flow are wheat bread, pasta, toast without jam, popcorn, and pretzels. But don't eat so many high-calorie foods that when you break into a smile with healthy teeth you've got a triple chin beneath them! Moderation is the key.

Now for some good news. It's been shown that chocolate's tannins and cocoa actually lessen the harmful effects of the sugar content. So, if you must, have a chocolate sweet, with meals, and brush afterward.

Although some artificial sweeteners don't cause cavities, some dentists say that sorbitol, if consumed to excess, may eventually cause decay.

Sugar is not your only enemy. People who like to suck on lemons (as I did when I was a child, with salt no less!) or who sip fruit juices and diet sodas all day long could be giving their teeth a continuous acid bath that eventually wears down enamel. If you need to sip a lot, it's better to dilute juices with seltzer water. You don't have to give up your citrus—you need the vitamin C—but I'm talking about people who sip all day long, not just at mealtime.

Fluoride in toothpaste and mouthwash have been proven protectors from tooth decay. If your city doesn't add fluoride to the water, see your dentist for advice about special fluoride treatments.

When you're out of toothpaste, dip your damp toothbrush in baking soda or a mixture of baking soda and salt, and brush. Add cloves if you want to spice up the flavor of your homemade toothpaste. Many dentists believe that regular brushing with baking soda and/ or salt is too abrasive for regular use. Find out what *your* dentist thinks next time you visit him.

• *THE RIGHT TOOTHBRUSH* •

Forget your toothbrush? Just put some toothpaste on your finger and "brush" away. I keep a toothbrush in my travel makeup kit so that I won't ever be without.

One of my readers came up with a solution for what to do if your toothbrush bristles are sprangled out. She wraps a twist-tie around the bottom of the wet toothbrush bristles, then pushes it up to the top. When the bristles are dry. they are back in the right shape. But don't use an old toothbrush too long. You could end up damaging your gums with sharp, broken bristles. Aren't the few dollars a year worth the investment?

The best toothbrush, dentists say, is a soft, multitufted brush in a size that fits into the corners of your mouth.

If you don't know if you're brushing properly, get some red disclosing tablets at the drugstore. Brush; chew the tablet; spit out the remains; look in a mirror to find the spots you've missed; brush them. This is a great way for children and some of us adults to see how well we really clean our teeth. But don't use a disclosing tablet before going out on a big date, you may end up looking like you have some horrible mouth disease!

• *HEALTHY GUMS* •

Pink gums are healthy gums. If yours are red, shiny, and if they bleed easily, you may have periodontal disease. Usually caused by poor cleansing habits, periodontal disease (gingivitis, pyorrhea) can eventually cause you to lose your teeth. Brush twice and floss once each day to keep the food debris and bacterial plaque from building up on your teeth and gums, and see your dentist as soon as possible if you have any of the signs of periodontal disease.

• *BAD BREATH* •

Bacterial growth in the mouth (also on the tongue) results in bad breath. When you brush your teeth, occasionally brush your tongue, too, or clean it by lightly scraping it with a spoon. Your tongue can be pink to coral or pinkish purple and still be healthy, but if it is whitish or yellowish, you may have a bacterial coating or a digestive problem. If, after cleaning your tongue, it still doesn't look healthy, see your physician.

• *MOUTH FRESHENERS* •

Not all mouth fresheners have to be bought at the drugstore; nor do they have to taste like medicine.

• *Parsley Plus:* yes, you heard right. Eat the parsley that garnishes your restaurant dinner. It's an old-fashioned breath cleanser and it's nutritious.

• *Leafy Tea:* try chewing fresh mint, or brew an herb tea (about two teaspoons mint, rosemary, thyme, or sage in about two cups of water), and then either drink the tea or keep in it your refrigerator for use as a mouthwash.

• *Ginger:* chop an ounce of ginger root; simmer in two cups of water for about fifteen minutes; strain; cool; store in fridge. Other spices, such as cloves, anise, and cinnamon sticks, can be made into mouth-freshener teas. Some may need to steep for thirty minutes or so to get full flavor, and you can mix and match flavors to get those you like.

• *DENTURES* •

You have to keep dentures clean to avoid bad breath. Baking soda works best. Brush it on; soak them in a glass of water with two teaspoons baking soda; rinse, and wear.

One of my readers carries a small piece of nylon net in her purse to use as a "brush" for quick cleanups of her dentures. This way, she can give her front teeth a quick scrub without having to remove them.

Another reader suggested that, while eating, you spear each bite-size piece of meat through the tine of the fork. Then, you will have four easily chewed pieces that still look like one piece. This will keep you from feeling as if you are cutting meat for a toddler.

When denture wearers get stuck with a hunk that just can't be chewed by a human being, it's better to find a way to get rid of the meat than to try to choke it down. Use your napkin; excuse yourself and go to the bathroom commode; whatever you do, get rid of it. It's easier to find a place to throw away a hunk of meat than it is to find someone to give you a Heimlich hug!

No one will deny that loose full or partial dentures can be embarrassing and can make eating a chore. Although liners and other aids for loose dentures can be purchased at the drugstore, the best way to solve the problem is to have the dentures refitted.

There are people who have difficulty getting dentures to fit properly. If you are one of these people, you may be a candidate for implant surgery, a procedure by which a device is inserted into or attached to the upper or lower jawbone. The implant, which can be inserted either at the time teeth are extracted or later, becomes anchored in the bone or attached to the bone. Full or partial dentures, bridges containing several teeth, or a single tooth can be attached to implants. You can eat normally, using your implants, as soon as three or four weeks after surgery; the recovery time depends on your healing and the type of implant used.

The problem with implants is that it's not easy to find a dentist who will perform them. Most older dentists are conservative and simply don't do them. Younger dentists, many of whom have had the training in dental school, graduate school, or at special courses, can't afford to invest in the implants and equipment unless enough patients ask for it. Only those trained in the technique should do them. To find a dentist in your area who is qualified to perform this surgery, call your local city or state dental society, or contact the American Academy of Implant Dentistry (AAID), 515 Washington Street, Avington, Massachusetts 02351.

• *EMERGENCY* •

If you get a tooth knocked out, the important thing is to keep the tooth moist. If it has not been cracked or fractured, gently put it back into the socket. If you are afraid to do this, simply rinse off the tooth (do *not* scrub or scrape it—that will remove the fibers that make it stay in place) and put the tooth in a moist tissue or cotton wad, or a container of milk or water. See a dentist immediately. The emphasis here is on protecting the tooth from damage and keeping it moist. If you can get to a dentist within several hours, you may be able to save your tooth.

A good book for you to read if you are considering any cosmetic dental work is *Change Your Smile* by Dr. Ronald E. Goldstein (Quintessence Publishing, Inc., 1984). It's worth the price of the book to learn all about dental work, so you know what to expect.

Chapter 6

HANDS UP! DO THEY PASS INSPECTION?

ou don't have to be a gypsy fortune teller to know that hands lead a tough life—and if you don't take care of them, it shows.

Everybody knows that the worst hangnails inevitably pop up when you need to look your best or are pulling on your most expensive pair of pantyhose, never when you are putting on multi-snagged, washed-out, bargain pantyhose. I certainly proved this when I went through three pairs of pantyhose in five minutes right before stepping onto the set for NBC's "Today Show."

Fingernails are composed of hornlike layers of dead cells held together by a substance called keratin. When detergents, chemicals, or other abuses destroy the keratin in your nails, they tend to split and break.

Creaming your hands and nails should be part of your beauty routine. Professional manicures and pedicures can be expensive, but you can learn to do them at home. Many dieters tell me they give themselves manicures and pedicures when they are about to succumb to munchies madness—it's hard to pick up high-calorie morsels when there's creamy goop on hands or wet polish on nails, and you can't get to the fridge when you have tissues or cotton wadded between your toes.

• *MANICURING YOUR NAILS* •

Remove old polish with a gentle polish remover. *Do not* peel off nail polish. I know it may be fun, but you will end up weakening the nail. I used to do this in my most boring math class in college, leaving behind a pile of polish on the desk. It didn't exactly endear me to the professor!

After removing polish, massage your hands, arms, and elbows with lotion, paying special attention to your cuticles and nails. Some people prefer to use creams and removers specially made for cuticles; I use any cream that softens the cuticles and I really enjoy soaking my hands and feet in warm, soapy water.

File your nails by holding the file vertically against the nail. Most people agree that filing in one direction—from edge to center—is best. Strive for a rounded or oval look. Filing too sharply at the edges of your nails (selvages) to create a pointed look weakens the sides and, some say, causes hangnails. Damaging the selvage of a nail also causes the nail to fan out. I file my nails to an almost square shape.

When you clean your fingernails with a file or orangewood stick tip, it's best to start at the corners and work to the center; then go under the center of the nail. If you work from the center to the corners, you'll push the dirt into the sides of your nails and damage the selvage.

Next, soak your fingers in warm, soapy water or a warm half vinegar–half water solution for five minutes. I like to apply glycerin to stubborn cuticles after soaking and before working to help push them back.

After soaking, *gently* push cuticles back with an orangewood stick wrapped in cotton or a cotton swab. Be especially gentle with the matrix (place from which your nails grow). If you damage the matrix, your nails will grow out with ridges or other deformities. And pressing too hard when pushing back your cuticles will cause horizontal ridges on the nail surface as it grows out. It takes about six months for damage to the matrix to heal and, until it heals, defects will occur in your nails as they grow.

It's okay to cut ragged, torn cuticles off with sharp, fine cuticle scissors *occasionally*, but regular cutting of the cuticle makes it tough and hard. Remember, it's the cuticle around the nail that holds it in place. When the cuticle is cut away or broken, the skin around the nails rolls back and causes hangnails.

• *CARE FOR CUTICLES, NAILS, AND HANDS* •

If you have problems with ragged cuticles or dry, chapped hands, try frequent treatments with petroleum jelly, olive or other oil. Before you go to bed at night, rub the petroleum jelly or oil into your hands, especially into your cuticles and nails, and then wear an old pair of cotton gloves to bed. If you don't have an old pair of cotton gloves, buy some—it's worth it. You can usually find relatively cheap all-cotton gloves in military or uniform stores or anyplace that stocks school marching band uniforms. These gloves are not particularly pretty, but quite washable and sturdy and, best of all, they're made of soft, absorbent cotton. I've used old socks or knee-highs, too.

You can also give your hands and nails a treatment when you wash dishes. Just apply cream, lotion, petroleum jelly, or other oil before you slip hands into cotton and over them rubber gloves. (One of my research assistants has used baby cream—not baby oil or lotion, although these work too—and says that though it's greasy because of the high lanolin content, it's very effective on hands and feet, cuticles and nails.)

Whatever you do to your cuticles and hangnails, don't bite them. And don't bite your fingernails either. But your mother probably told you that years ago. I was a nail biter up until seventh grade. What cured me? The boy I had a tremendous crush on grabbed my hand and said, "Who wants to hold hands with *that* ugly hand?" Since then, I have made every effort to take care of my hands and nails. How I wish I would run into that boy now!

If you do bite your nails, manicuring and polishing them regularly can be a really effective cure for the nasty habit. It's certainly worth a try, and the bonus is pretty hands that you don't have to hide in your pockets.

• *WORK GLOVES* •

Rubber gloves protect your hands and nails. If your skin is sensitive to the rubber, sprinkle powder—baby, talc, cornstarch—into the gloves and wear cotton gloves inside the rubber ones. Even if your skin is not sensitive to the rubber, the gloves will slip off and on more easily if you put some sort of powder in them. They'll *feel* better, too.

• WEATHER OR NOT •

Did you know that climate can dry out your nails and make them brittle? In cold or very dry weather, be sure to moisturize your nails to prevent cracking, peeling, and breaking. Wear nail polish to harden and protect nails, and when you remove it use a low-acetone remover to prevent drying out the nails. Some experts recommend removing polish entirely every few weeks just to let your nails "breath" for about a week, as a problem-prevention measure.

• HARDENING NAILS •

Remember the old wives' tale about eating or drinking gelatin to make strong nails? Well it's not exactly yummy stuff when mixed in water. Although gelatin may be good for salad or dessert, recent research indicates that it's the protein in your diet—not the gelatin —that makes your nails strong and healthy. I know someone who swears that her nails get stronger a few months after she begins one of her daily doses of yogurt-for-health diets. Yogurt *is* high in protein, so she could be right.

Nail hardeners are available at cosmetic counters, but many of them contain formaldehyde, a chemical that can cause adverse reactions. Try using these products on one nail only for about a week to test for problems before you paint them on all of your nails.

One inexpensive nail hardener available at your friendly pharmacy is white iodine. It's cheap and can prevent flaking and peeling. Put the iodine on your nails every night for one week, then once a week or less often just to maintain hardness. You don't want to do it too often because it may make your nails too hard and brittle. Nails need to be somewhat flexible. And by the way, if you are treating your nails with white iodine, don't let them come into contact with peroxide or they might turn orange!

For hard but flexible nails try moisturizing them frequently with glycerin, cream, lotion, petroleum jelly, or oils.

And don't forget that prevention is easier than cure. Use a pencil or pen to dial the phone or press buttons. Use a "church key" bottle opener, screwdriver, putty knife, or metal spatula to pry up lids—not your thumbnail. I've even learned to use my knuckle when hitting a push-button phone!

· MIX AND MATCH ·

I thought I knew almost everything about nail care—I've been painting my nails since I was fourteen years old. When I think of all the time I've spent looking for just the right shade of red or something with a little less pink, or a bronze to go with a new suit, and then had to settle for whatever was on the shelf, I just wish that my friend had given me this hint sooner.

Here's what she does and what I do now: I take an empty bottle I've saved and cleaned, and line up all the colors I have. Then I play mix and match.

I start with the color that's closest to what I want—let's say a deep red—then I add another color to make it a little lighter, or more pink-toned, or I may even add a dash of gold. Since I've been mixing my own, I've had more fun, and best of all, I've been able to get the "just right" shades I've wanted from the polish I already have. Test your custom color on a toenail or a white sheet of paper. You'll want to put down some paper towels or newspapers before you start mixing polishes, because it can get messy.

· MORE POLISHING POINTERS ·

Here are some other polishing tips. The professionals apply a clear or base coat (you'll find some called "filler" that help cover up ridges) and then two coats of color, and a final sealing coat. When you put on the sealer, don't stop at the edge of your nail; paint over and under the edge for a real seal to your color. And for extra seal, put a layer of sealer or clear polish on, extended over and under the edge of your nail the day after a manicure.

I like to dip a small piece of cotton in vinegar (yes, it's that wonderful vinegar again!) and wipe each nail. When I use a deep red polish on long nails, I start polishing by doing the tip of the nail first, then start at the base and polish over the entire nail. This seems to add more with only one coat where my nails need it most, on the tips, where they seem to chip first.

· SMUDGE REMOVAL ·

Don't you just hate it when you slip a bit while polishing your nails and polish on the skin beside your nails? Here's how the pros solve that clean-up problem. Dip a wooden toothpick into polish remover, wrap cotton thread around the end, dip in remover again, and you have a fine tool for getting those tiny blots and smears without disturbing your nails at all. A cotton swab works, too, but you can't get as close to the nail as you can with the toothpick.

The easiest solution for folks who, no matter how they try, can't seem to get polish on neatly is to use clear or natural-color polish.

· STORAGE TIPS ·

And while we're talking about nail polish, I wonder how I could have overlooked the simplest solution to mixing polish for as long as I did. You know the kind of polish that has the white stuff that always settles to the bottom? Usually, just to get it mixed well enough to use, you have to shake and shake until you lose all interest in polishing your nails. I finally learned to store polish bottles on their sides, so the white stuff settles to the bottle's side, and mixing it with the brush is a snap.

Here's another one of those, "Why didn't I think of this sooner" ideas. One of my readers suggested greasing the treads of nail polish bottle caps with petroleum jelly to keep the caps from sticking to the bottles. Some folks unstick caps from polish bottles by putting them in the microwave for a second, or running them under hot water.

Always screw those caps back on tightly to keep your polish from drying out, but if it should get dry or too thick, just thin out your nail polish with some enamel solvent or nail polish remover; give the bottle a shake, and then you'll be able to use your favorite polish to the very last drop. Thin polish makes a better surface and dries better and faster when you put on two to three coats. But thick, old polish is good when you only have time for one coat.

Here's how to speed up drying your nail polish: wait a few minutes, then dip your nails into a bowl of ice water.

I like to dot each nail with a drop of safflower or other vegetable oil a few minutes after a manicure.

• *REPAIRS FOR BROKEN NAILS* •

You can buy kits for repairing your nails with plastic "caps," and some have an adhesive paper you can use to wrap your nails. Wrapping is considered by most experts to be the best protection for problem nails. Wrap according to directions and then polish. Be patient—it takes practice to get it right.

A quick repair for a ripped or broken nail is quick-drying glue, but take care when using those instant-drying glues—if you're not too handy, you can end up gluing your fingers together. *Always* use solvents (those made specifically for the glue, acetone, or nail polish remover) to remove fast-drying glues. *Never* use razor blades to separate your fingers from each other or you may end up in the emergency room.

If you're all thumbs and don't want to glue your hand into a mitten shape, you might have better luck using the kind of cement that is used to repair china or jewelry.

If your tear or break needs reinforcement, such as a tear halfway across your nail (and don't you just get goose bumps thinking about it?), you can make your own repair kit with some quick-drying glue or china or jewelry cement and thin paper—cigarette papers, part of an unused tea bag, a piece of your coffeepot filter. Tear a small patch of the paper (so the fibers will be tapered at the edges) to a size that's as wide as the nail break and about a half an inch long. First, glue the nail tear together and let dry. Next, saturate the patch with glue or cement, then weave it around the torn nail, gluing part of the paper to the body of the nail, and folding the paper around the torn part and in back across the top of the torn part. Smooth the paper fringes down with cement and an orangewood stick or the side of a toothpick. Use a second patch if necessary. Be careful not to glue either of the patches to your skin. Smooth the patch with an orangewood stick or the side of a toothpick, and after it's all dry, cover with several base coats and a few coats of nail polish.

· QUICK-FIX TIPS ·

Don't throw away your emery boards when the edges are worn right down the middle. Cut them in half and you'll have two good sides for filing your nails.

Stains around the cuticles and those little crevices on your fingers and elbow can be removed in a flash—or rather a rub. Put a dab of cuticle remover on a piece of cotton and massage away; then rinse.

You can't fix those little white spots that show up on your nails. They are caused by bruises and air bubbles in the nail's body and you'll just have to wait for them to grow out. Friends tell me that in some parts of the country, children say that the number of white spots on your fingernails tells the number of boy or girl friends you have. Guess they aren't all that bad to have!

Chapter 7

YOUR FEET: THEY NEED PAMPERING TOO

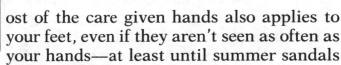

ost of the care given hands also applies to your feet, even if they aren't seen as often as your hands—at least until summer sandals reveal whatever's been neglected all winter.

Polish removal, cuticle care, massage with softening agents, soaking, and polish application are all much like hand care, but feet need extra care for dry skin and calluses. If you pumice away dry skin and apply some sort of lotion or cream daily, you aren't likely to need a major conditioning; but if you've neglected your feet, you will need to work at getting them back to their baby softness, especially on your heels and the balls of your feet. A pumice stone will be kinder to your skin if you wet and soap it up before rubbing it on your dry skin and calluses.

When filing your toenails, it's best to clip and file them straight across to avoid ingrown toenails. Clipping them when they are wet softens them. Polish your toenails using the same method as you did with your fingernails, and if you are planning a weekend at the beach, your toenails won't look so chipped and scruffy from kicking up your toes in the sand if you use a natural or light shade of polish. When polishing your toenails, you can separate your toes with cotton balls or a tissue or toilet tissue rolled and woven up and down through the spaces between your toes.

If your toes, nails, or the skin on your feet are discolored, rub the discolored areas with half a lemon, which you can cup on your heels for fifteen minutes for extra bleaching and softening; then put the same lemon "caps" on your elbows.

If you plug the drain in your tub when you take a shower, you can soak your feet while you shower.

· KINDNESS TO YOUR FEET ·

After bathing or showering, dry your feet well and dust them with foot, talc, or other powder to keep them comfy, dry, and fungus-free. Also avoid fungus by wearing beach sandals when showering in public facilities. Avoid powders with starch in them; starch feeds bacteria, which can cause odors.

When you have tired, achy feet, try sitting at the edge of the tub and alternating running cold and hot water on your feet for a few "rounds," or set up two basins—one with hot and one with ice water—in the tub and alternate dipping your feet in them. Doing this in the tub is less messy than putting two basins on the floor.

Overheated feet in the summer? Try spraying them with a light cologne; the alcohol will cool them off. Or just dab your feet with an alcohol-dipped cotton ball. When you're traveling and touring, you can freshen your feet by dabbing at them with a moist towelette—even through your pantyhose.

A good exercise for tired, achy feet is to roll them over a can or pop bottle, and don't forget how good a massage with lotion can make your feet feel.

Another exercise is a wall walk. Lie flat on the floor, arms at your sides, and then walk up the wall and prop your feet and legs up on the wall for about five minutes.

To prevent foot problems, you really shouldn't wear shoes that give you corns, calluses, or pain. And remember that your socks and panty hose should be half an inch longer than your big toe.

You are less likely to buy pain-producing shoes if you shop in the late afternoon. Why? Your feet are larger in late afternoon (from water retention), so you're more likely to get a better fit.

I still chuckle at the question one of my readers asked several years ago: "When your feet hurt, all you have to do is take off your shoes. So when your head hurts, will it help if you take off your hat?"

Let's hope neither your feet nor your head hurt very often.

Chapter 8

MAKEUP: THE BEAUTY YOU GIVE YOURSELF

M akeup can cover almost any beauty flaw, and when applied well, it accents your best features. Of course, it can't substitute for good health, good grooming, and a positive attitude—but it helps.

Don't let the price tag determine what makeup products you buy. Rather, choose the makeup that will work best for your skin type and your life-style. Study the ingredients. You'll soon find that cosmetics on both ends of the price range are formulated with many of the same ingredients. And very often what you're paying for with all those fancy, expensive creams is the advertising, promotion, and packaging. Plain old mineral oil keeps your skin just as smooth as a brand-named moisturizer or hormone cream—and it costs much, much less. But people are easily fooled. Consumer-group surveys of cosmetic users reveal that, in general, consumers rate more expensive brands of liquid foundation and mascara higher for consistency and durability.

You have to find the cosmetics that work best for you. Here are some tips I've developed myself or learned from my readers and professional cosmetologists.

• *THE RIGHT LIGHT* •

Whenever you put on makeup, be sure to apply it in the kind of light it will be viewed in. For example, if you're going to be spending the day outdoors, check yourself out in the mirror next to the window. Beware of overhead lights; they can distort the way your makeup looks.

If you're going out in the evening to a dimly lit restaurant, you will need more color and definition than usual. But don't go overboard!

I carry a purse emergency makeup kit with miniatures of things I can use, which really comes in handy when I want to touch up my makeup so that it's right for the lighting, wherever I am. See the emergency makeup kit list later in this chapter.

I can't stress enough the importance of making sure your daytime makeup is right for daylight and your nighttime makeup is right for artificial night light. Sparkling, shining eye shadows really aren't for daytime wear—they make you look like a disco queen or a Las Vegas showgirl. During the daytime, be sure the makeup you wear is appropriate for the setting and circumstances.

It's pretty easy to slip into a routine in the way you present yourself to the world. I catch myself forgetting that there really is a difference between night and day. What is called a "natural look" can be fine, and you can add a bit more to natural as long as you watch what and how much you add. Save those shiny golds and silvers for a special sparkly nighttime look. Aim to look natural in the daytime and fantastic at night.

I firmly believe that the purpose of makeup is to minimize or conceal flaws—not to make you look painted. To avoid this, make sure you see your face from all angles as you apply makeup—the sides when you are applying blush, for example, so that you don't end up with two round circles on your cheeks.

Nor do you want a distinct line where your foundation ends at your chin or jawline—especially if you are using a foundation color that is slightly darker than your skin's natural tone. I blend my foundation around my chin and neck with a clean sponge, or pat it on lightly with a facial tissue. If you use a cover stick under your eyes or on facial blemishes, pat it on your skin—never rub. This way the cover-up will do its job more effectively.

This is also true of foundation, especially if you have large pores or scars from acne, etc. I have a few spots that I pat my foundation over, and then I go over these spots once more to really cover them. I don't mean you should apply heavy coats of cover-up—all you need is enough to make a foundation for your foundation.

I use a big brush or a facial tissue to blend rouge or blusher so that it looks natural.

When you are putting on makeup for a black-and-white photograph, apply a little more blusher than usual. Use a lip brush to get a more defined mouth outline. Don't use frosted lip color. Just before going in front of the camera, dust your face lightly with powder; most pros use a translucent powder.

• BUYING AND STORING COSMETICS •

According to the manufacturers, when cosmetics cause problems, it's because of misuse by consumers. Exposure to extreme cold, heat, or light, for example, shortens the shelf life of most cosmetics. Most cosmetics that have been opened are good for a year, unless they have been contaminated by the consumer; most manufacturers say products should definitely not be kept longer than two or three years, even with proper storage.

Here are some recommendations from the experts:

• If the package has been opened, or appears tampered with, do not buy the product, whatever the price.

• If, after you open a product, you discover that it has a strange odor, seems dried out, or just doesn't look right, return it.

• Apply cosmetics to a clean face with a clean hand, and keep containers tightly closed, to prevent contamination.

• Mix one "dose" at a time. For example, if you are combining two shades of foundation, mix what you need for a single application in your palm instead of pouring the contents of one container into the other. Another reason for not mixing more than one dose is that the color you create may not be what you want and you'll have messed up two bottles of foundation instead of just a palmful.

Of course, if you have only a little bit left in each container, I don't think you need to worry about contamination because what you've mixed will be used up quickly. I mix my own colors with all of my cosmetics.

• When testing sample cosmetics in stores, apply the products on the palms of your hands, *never* on your lips or eyes.

• Never use cosmetics on broken or irritated skin; especially avoid putting cosmetics on sores or rashes caused by varicose veins.

• Don't *share* cosmetics. Sharing can cause different types of bacteria to mingle, resulting in a variety of infections. Some experts say that it's possible to transmit herpes virus by sharing lipsticks. That's also the reason you shouldn't use store testers on your lips or eyes—lest you invite infections caused by germs or viruses left behind by other users.

• Don't store cosmetics on windowsills, radiator tops, or in your car during hot weather; excessive light from sun or artificial sources, heat, or cold can cause them to deteriorate rapidly. The exceptions are creams and lotions, which last longer if stored in the refrigerator. During the summer, many people like to keep their astringents or skin fresheners in the refrigerator for an extra perk.

• Eye products have their own sets of rules. If you are allergy-prone, keep eye products for only three to four months. If, for example, you accidentally scratch the cornea of your eye while applying mascara, bacteria from your eye can get into the tube and contaminate it. Even if you're not allergy-prone, the professionals advise getting a new mascara every six months, because containers older than that can carry bacteria and, therefore, may cause infection. Aren't your eyes worth $2 to $5 every six months? (For more about eyes, go to the section in this chapter on eye makeup.)

• Fragrances don't last forever. They oxidize, which changes the balance of oils and alcohol, and they evaporate. (For more on fragrances, go to Chapter 9.)

• MAKEUP INGREDIENTS—LEARN A FEW NEW WORDS •

If you have sensitive skin, keep in mind that fewer ingredients in your cosmetics means fewer chemicals to irritate your skin.

Colognes, astringents, and aftershaves containing oil of bergamot or extract of lemon, orange, or lime may make your skin sensitive to sun, causing rashes or burns that leave discolored patches even *after* the irritation has healed. Other common irritants are quaternium 15 or formaldehyde, often used as preservatives in fragrances; isopropyl myristate, which makes skin more absorbent to irritating chemicals; propylene glycol, a common humectant (water-attracting agent) found in moisturizers.

Cosmetics to look for are those listing among their ingredients hydrophilic ointment USSP, urea, and mineral oil. You can tell if a product is hydrophilic (combined with water, as is recommended by dermatologists) by putting some of the product in your palm, adding a few drops of water, and rubbing. If the liquid disappears easily, the product is hydrophilic.

Generally, preservatives need to be added to cosmetics to prevent bacteria from growing in them and spoiling them. Emulsifiers are necessary to keep products creamy and spreadable. But most perfumes, colorings, and thickeners merely make products more expensive when they are added and aren't really necessary.

• *MAKEUP CHANGES* •

If you're like me, you probably get stuck from time to time in a beauty routine, just because it's simple and convenient. If you like the way you look, then by all means, stick with it. But if you think that you would like to make small changes, or look a little different, think about your makeup and take a close look at your "finished" face. Sometimes a change as subtle as the color of your mascara or blush or a different placement for your eyeliner can create a whole new look.

Beware of trends. If you are wearing a look that was popular or in many years ago, you're dating yourself and will look older.

Sometimes it's wise to change your makeup, even if it looks great. Occasionally, manufacturers change their formulas, so that an "old faithful" product can turn into an irritant; also, your body chemistry changes, turning a product you've used forever into one you have to avoid. It's happened to me and when I finally called the manufacturer to ask, I learned that my old faithful had a new formula.

Don't dismiss dime-store makeup—it can come in very handy when you want to make a change. Remember, you don't *have* to spend a bundle and run the risk of ending up with a look you may not like.

Check out drug stores and dime stores for samples of foundation, shampoo, conditioners, sprays, deodorants, and fragrances. Look for sale bins filled with shelf-worn items. It doesn't matter if the label is scraped or the outer box is missing, as long as the bottle hasn't been opened.

Very often it's the undesirable items—odd-colored lipsticks and liners, unusual shades of eyeshadows—that are marked more than half off. Although at first you may dismiss them, you *can* mix your own lipstick colors and end up with exactly the shade you want— at a bargain price! Sale bins also give you a chance to try types of makeup you haven't used before—like loose powder instead of pressed, cream instead of powdered blusher, and so forth.

Wander around department-store makeup sections and check out the freebies. You may be able to get one of the best freebies of all— a free makeover from a cosmetic house representative. Now, I know that this could make you feel guilty—taking up somebody's time and free makeup when you don't intend to purchase anything—but think of it this way: you have helped the cosmetician by volunteering as a free model for the demonstration. Not *everybody* has the nerve to get made up while strangers watch. If you really feel guilty, buy the smallest size of the cheapest item sold to clear your conscience.

· FDA HELP ·

If you have problems with makeup—you don't understand the directions, or the label is misleading—complain to the Food and Drug Administration, Division of Cosmetics Technology, HFF-430, 200 C Street S.W., Washington D.C. 20204.

· FOUNDATION: THE BASE ·

It's said that makeup can't cover up your personality or your character, but it sure can cover up a lot of other things, and that's why it's important to choose the right color for your foundation or makeup base. It will restructure feature flaws and blend color variations of your skin and in general will give your skin a smoother appearance.

Test for Color

When you test for color at the cosmetics counter, don't rub the product on your palm or wrist—the skin tones are usually not the same as your face. Instead, use the skin of your jaw; then you can see how the color blends with the skin tone of your neck. I like to use the back of my hand when color testing too. If you choose the proper color, then you won't have to put makeup on your neck, where it will rub off and ruin your clothing. You can just blend your makeup base over the edge of your jaw, the way the experts say you should.

Here's a good hint: ivory or neutral-colored foundations help to disguise redness at the base of the nose or of tiny broken blood vessels on the face.

Keep this in mind, too: there's no rule that says you can't mix several shades of foundation in the palm of your hand to get the right color for your skin. Mixing your own single dose of foundation may be just what you'll need to do if you've been outdoors and have just enough of a tan to alter your normal skin tone, so that your usual foundation doesn't quite match. (Remember, experts advise that mixing cosmetics in their containers can cause contamination; that's why it's best to mix one dose in the palm of your hand.)

Skin Types

Women with dry skin should use an oil-based foundation; women with oily skin should use a water-based or emulsion-type foundation, which contains little or no oil. Women blessed with normal skin can choose just about any kind of foundation, and those with combination skin (oily and dry patches) will find some foundations on the market designed especially for them. Or they may need to experiment with different types of foundations before they find the one that works for them.

You may be one of those people who needs to use different makeup bases during different seasons of the year. For example, if winter dries your skin, you may need oil-based makeup on those frosty early February days; and if summer heat causes excess oiliness, you may need water-based makeup.

Which Foundations Last the Longest?

Cream foundations, usually sold in small pots or compacts, last the longest. Second longest are oil-in-water emulsions. Water-based foundations last the least amount of time. Women with oily skin usually think creams feel too heavy; you can mix equal parts of oil-based and water-based foundations in the palms of your hands before applying.

Applying Foundation

Before applying foundation, you should cleanse, tone, and moisturize according to your skin type. See the section on skin types. Most of the experts suggest applying foundation with a moist sponge to avoid that mask look and to get a better blend across your skin.

Here's a good trick for putting foundation on evenly: dot foundation—and I mean dot, not blob (less is more)—on your chin, cheeks, outer corners of your mouth, under your nose, under each eye, and on each lid, with three or four dots on your forehead. Swirl the dots around to blend on your face and over your jawline with a damp or dry sponge, cotton ball, or makeup square. (For advice on how to make your own wedge makeup sponges, go to the substitutions section of this chapter.) Sometimes I use a lighter foundation just under my eye area and blend well. This lightens but doesn't give the raccoon look that comes from using a highlighter.

Waterproof/Water-Resistant

Water-resistant means that the makeup won't streak or run in the humidity or when you perspire. Water-resistant makeup *will* wipe off with a towel or tissue, but otherwise you can expect water-resistant makeup to last about six to eight hours—whether it's in misty rain or while you're sweating.

Waterproof makeup isn't supposed to come off at all—either when wet *or* rubbed. At a major cosmetics firm, waterproof products must pass the swimming pool test: they must stay on during a half hour of swimming.

Waterproof/water-resistant makeups usually have a high oil content and are generally *not* suited to oily skin.

Making Makeup Last Longer on Your Skin

No matter how you put it on or what kind of makeup you use, cosmetologists say you can't expect your makeup to stay picture perfect for more than six hours—even if you choose the right kind for your skin type and apply it properly. But here are some tips.

Loose or pressed powder brushed or patted on with a puff, sets makeup. Take a sponge that's been dampened with cool water and dab it over your powder to get a glow on your skin. Instead of cool water, some women like to use a sponge or cotton ball dipped in mild astringent lotion to set makeup after the powder has been applied.

The area around your eyes will have a moister look if you don't powder it.

Keep your powder dry! If you use loose powder, store it in an old salt or pepper shaker so you can pour just as much as you need on your palm, then dip a makeup brush (or puff if you prefer) into the powder and dust it on.

Save those old blush brushes for powder! Or use a shaving brush. One of my friends "borrowed" her husband's shaving brush, and she says it's the greatest.

• *EYE MAKEUP* •

One thing I've learned from my friends is that some of the lash-lengthening mascaras contain little fibers than can flake off and get into your eyes. If your eyes burn or itch from any eye product, stop using it!

Be careful with eye shadows, too. As I've mentioned, some of the iridescent shiny shadows contain such ingredients as ground-up pearl, and when flecks of these shadows fall into your eyes, they can cause problems, too.

Have you ever noticed how you can almost change your eye color with eyeshadow? For example, I have a blue-eyed friend, whose eyes almost look violet when she wears purple shadow and/or purple clothing.

Some beauty experts say you shouldn't wear eye shadow that's the same color as your eyes. I think you should wear whatever color you like, but remember that what you wear during the day should not be what you wear at night. Keep it soft and subtle for day unless you want to look like a punk rocker or a disco queen. Save the dramatic looks for after dark.

As always when you apply or blend any kind of makeup around your eyes, take care not to abuse the delicate area around your eyes. Gently, use either a cotton swab or your fingers. When you use your fingers, always use your ring fingers, the ones next to your pinkies. Never use your index or middle fingers—they are apt to exert too much pressure. You hardly use your ring finger to do anything, therefore it's weaker and will be more gentle to the tissue around your eyes.

If you apply moisturizer to the eye area before putting makeup on, then let it set for a while before starting. You won't have to work so hard to blend the concealers, shadows, and so forth. Be kind to your eyes!

Eye Sculpture

If you know how, you can almost sculpture a new look with eye shadows and eye makeup techniques. Here's how the experts make eyes look more important.

ENLARGING SMALL EYES Apply light, neutral shadow from your lashes to your brow; put a medium tone on your lid, and outline the outer two-thirds of your lids, drawing slightly larger outlines of your eyes on the outer corners, being careful not to try to go to an extreme. Blend all the lines and contours with a cotton-tipped swab. Apply gray or light brown mascara.

BRINGING OUT DEEP-SET EYES The idea here is to make the crease you have above your eye seem higher. Apply a light shade of foundation or cover stick on your eyelid and brow bone. Then blend a darker shade of the same foundation or concealer just above the crease of your eye. Put highlighter color just below the arch of your eyebrow. Blend all together. Line your lower eyelid with pencil and use lots of mascara—at least three coats.

WIDENING CLOSE-SET EYES Color is the key here. Use light, neutral eyeshadow if you have small, close-set eyes, and use darker colors for large, close-set eyes. You'll be putting the darker tones of concealer or shadow toward the outer two-thirds of your eye to make them seem wider-set. Begin by putting the lightest shadow on your eyelids, extending it to the brow bone. Then brush the medium tone of shadow on the outer upper two-thirds of your top and bottom lashes and, when you apply mascara, give several coats to the outer two-thirds of your lashes.

BALANCING PROTRUDING EYES Protruding eyes can look large, the way you want them to look, without protruding. Color is the trick here, as in all shading. Begin by putting a light to medium tone of eye shadow on the area from lashes to brow. Apply a darker tone on your eyelids below the crease. Dot highlighter at your eyebrow arch's highest point. Blend tones. Apply eyeliner beneath lower lashes. When you put on your mascara (use a dark tone), put most of the mascara right above your iris (the center).

Eye Colors

When it comes to choosing eye color, play around with various colors to see what looks best on you at different times of the day and with different colors of clothing. Here are some suggestions:

• *Blue-eyed Colors:* pale tints lighter than your eye color will make your eye color appear deeper. Try shades of gray with pink highlighters. Blue-eyed women can wear brown, gray, or blue eyeliner.

• *Green-eyed Colors:* contrasting violet can accent green eyes. So can a lime and yellow-gold combination of shadows. And try a navy eyeliner.

• *Hazel-eyed Colors:* key are the flecks of yellow-gold, green, and brown that are in hazel eyes. Shadows in beige, brown, and green work well. Pick up colors from the iris for all eye makeup.

• *Brown-eyed Colors:* gray or purple shadow complements brown eyes. Pencil can be very dark black, blue, purple, or brown.

• *Black-eyed Colors:* black, charcoal, and pale gray or mauve, as well as pale pink, will accent black eyes.

Makeup shades change each season, but some rules always apply. Lighter, more subtle, and natural colors are more appropriate for the daytime, and the more exotic look is better suited to night. Eye makeup under glasses can be a little more dramatic so that your eyes aren't hidden while they are helped to see! You can always do one eye first to see if you like the effect.

Eye Dos

Here are some hints:

• Conceal under-eye shadows with concealer in a shade that's lighter than skin tone.

• Shadow clings better and lasts longer if you dust it with translucent powder or baby powder.

• Apply cream eye shadow, followed by dusting of powder, and dusting of powdered eye shadow for long-lasting effects.

• Some experts say powdered shadows look better longer than creams, and that creams tend to "melt" into the folds of your eyelids. Powdered shadows will go on more smoothly if applied with a damp cosmetic sponge.

• If you don't like to use eye shadow but want to subtly accent your eyes, try using an eyeliner brush to draw a thin line of brown or gray cake shadow along the crease of your eyelid. Blend this line to softness *in* the crease, not up or down.

• Try mixing your own shadow shade by blending together several shades that complement your natural eye color.

Eyeliner Tips

If you want eyeliner to look good, never just draw a line, especially on the bottom lid. It looks too obvious and harsh. (Remember Cleopatra?) When you use liquid eyeliner, dot it on, starting at the outer corner of your eye. Dot, dot, dot along the lash line, in between the lashes, and it will look so much better than a hard line.

Here are some other eyeliner tips:

• Liquid eyeliner lasts longest, but many women still prefer crayon or pencil for lining their eyes. Eye crayon or pencil can be blended with cotton swabs for a softer look.

• To make pencil eyeliner look better and keep it from smearing, especially on the lower lid, some professional makeup artists apply all makeup, then put on pencil liner, powdering it to set it. The last step is to take a cotton swab, dust away excess powder, and slightly smudge the line so it doesn't look obvious.

• When you look as tired as you feel, it's a good idea not to put dark liner on your upper eyelid. It will only make you look sleepier.

Try lining only the outer half of your upper and lower lashes in gray or brown.

• When you don't feel up to putting on makeup, but need to add accent to your eyes for daytime, try applying a moisturizer to eyes and then outlining with a gray, light brown, or beige-toned pencil.

Mascara Tips

You've read about my mascara method in Chapter 1, "Strictly Personal." Here are some others:

• **Make sure your eyelashes are totally dry before applying mascara.**

• **When wearing false lashes, apply mascara on both false and natural lashes after the false ones are glued on for a more natural, blended look.**

• **Put mascara on the top (meaning from the upper lid out) and bottom of lashes of your upper and lower lids to get the best effect. Often the tops of your lashes are bleached a bit from the sun, and if you just put color on the bottoms of lashes you don't get a good, thick look.**

• **Try different mascara applicators to find which works best for you—straight or curved brushes, sponges, combs, wands, or flexible wands. Watch for mascaras specially made for sensitive eyes or for women who wear contact lenses.**

• **Buy a new mascara every six months. Old mascara can contain bacteria that may cause eye infections.**

• **Most women can wear dark brown or dark gray mascara. Jet black is for me!**

• **Powder lashes before applying mascara; apply mascara and another dusting of powder; add another application of mascara for a real accent to eyes; comb lashes with lash brush, comb, or toothbrush to keep them separate as you apply mascara layers.**

• **Your eyelash curler won't get gunky if you curl your eyelashes *before* you use mascara, instead of after.**

• **The ingredients in waterproof or water-resistant mascaras may sting eyes, even when these products are labeled hypoallergenic. If your eyes sting from one brand of mascara, try other brands until you find the one that suits your body chemistry. Some products will sting at first and then be comfortable after a few minutes. Testing is the only way to discover what suits you. Save the labels** to keep track. Some detective work on your part may provide clues to ingredients for you to avoid in *any* product.

• If you have a problem with mascara smudging on your lower lashes, apply only to your top lashes. I never wear mascara on my lower lashes because my eyes tear when I laugh—and I laugh a lot. Find what works for you and then use it to create your own look.

• Most experts say blondes should avoid black mascara because there's too much contrast; it makes them look tough. I say, who knows?

• When you don't feel like wearing makeup but want to show off eyes, apply a smidgen of petroleum jelly to your lids and lashes. It's good for your skin as a moisturizer and it conditions your lashes too. Petroleum jelly is an old-fashioned eyelash darkener, and many of my friends remember their mothers using it on them before they were old enough to wear makeup.

Eyebrows

See the section on eyebrows in Chapter 4 of this book.

Eye Makeup that Camouflages

Some women draw attention away from dark circles under the eyes by applying a cover-up stick in a shade that's lighter than their skin and foundation, just *below* the circles. Then they apply foundation. This way the lighter area on the cheekbone below the circles distracts from the circles.

Others prefer to use concealer in a shade lighter than skin, blending it on the upper lids, from the lash to the brow. Apply the appropriate color of eye shadow, then the mascara. It's important to blend the different tones of concealers with brush, cotton swab, or makeup sponge so they look natural. Always blend gently on the sensitive eye area.

Here are some other camouflage secrets:

• Cover puffy eyes with concealer two shades *darker* than your skin tone, using a brush or sponge to apply. Don't *ever* use white or very light concealer—it will accent puffy eyes.

• Diminish fine lines under eyes by applying a mixture of half foundation and half moisturizer. Pat mixture on gently. Roll a fine makeup sponge lightly back and forth over the area to blot up excess; dust with fine pressed matte powder to set.

• Crow's feet can also be diminished. Brush a very small amount of pale pressed powder on crow's feet to lighten the dark areas of the wrinkles. Then put most of your eye shadow in the area toward the center of your eye, to detract from the lines. Avoid getting shadow on crow's feet because it tends to accent them by darkening the creases. Lighter powder is also good to help hide wrinkles around the mouth.

• Don't forget how well tinted eyeglass lenses work as cover-ups and beauty enhancers. Gradient tints make your eyes look bigger, and rosy, peachy, amber, and warm brownish shades can put a healthy glow on your skin.

• *LIPS* •

According to a psychological study, people with full lips are thought to be happier looking, whereas people with thin lips are thought to be less cheery. Whether or not lips signal to everyone what your state of mind is, you can, if you want, change their fullness by slightly changing the outline around your lips. Of course, you don't want to go to extremes and make clown lips, but if you think your lips are too full, line them inside the lip line. If you think you need fuller lips, line them outside the lip line.

If you are not changing the outline of your lips, draw an M on your upper lip and then line your bottom lip from each corner to the center. After lining, fill in the color. For best results, use a lip brush.

Unlike the rest of your makeup, which is coordinated with your own personal coloring, lip color is usually chosen to correspond with the colors of clothing you're wearing.

Most women have a choice of several flattering shades of lipstick. Almost anyone can wear true red tones in lipsticks or lip glosses, but the general color rule is that fair-skinned women wear pink tones, and sallow-skinned women wear peach and brown tones. Your skin chemistry can alter the lipstick shades you wear, so you can't choose a color because it looks good on somebody else.

For a more natural look, your lipstick, like the rest of your makeup, should be subtle in bright daylight or harsh office light.

I always have the right color with me wherever I go because I keep blobs of lipstick of several different shades in a small compact —the kind that some lip glosses come in. My husband doesn't approve (he thinks it looks gross) but I know it's practical. You can also store them in a rouge container.

Then I use my lip brush to dip into the blob I want. This is also a good way to use up all those smidgens of lipstick left in the bottom of the tube. Just dip out the leftovers with a toothpick and make up your own custom colors compact.

When you are using up the leftovers in the bottom of a tube, you also have a chance to experiment and mix up a new custom shade. What can you lose? If you were going to throw away the leftovers anyway, a mess up of the colors is no loss. But most of the time, it won't be a mess up—it'll be another way to save some money.

Some Lip-Coloring Tricks

• If your lipstick tends to run or disappear, try applying foundation and face powder to your lips *before* you apply lipstick.

• Your lipstick will stay on longer if you apply it, blot, dab on powder, then reapply.

• Some women like to put on lipstick, blot, and apply clear gloss to protect the color and make it stay on longer.

• If untinted gloss or flesh-colored lipstick just doesn't do it for you, but you don't want to wear a true red lipstick, try outlining your lips with a lip pencil in a cherry or natural red before applying untinted gloss or flesh-colored lipstick. The bit of color from the lip liner showing through the gloss will define the shape of your lips and accent your mouth with a subtle, natural look instead of a lipstick-red look.

• If you don't like lip liner to be obvious, match your lip liner to your lipstick. Just put a line of each on your palm when you are testing the colors at the store to see if they match or blend.

• To accent your lips, try putting light brown eyebrow pencil in the corners of your mouth—*just* at the corners, not on the outside.

• Another accent is to place a dot of white in the center of your lips after you have outlined them with pencil, and then fill in as usual with color.

• If you can find a theatrical makeup supplier, the kabuki cake red that actors use around their eyes can also be painted on your lips—just like a watercolor—with a brush that's been dipped in water. This red will last all day, even through meals.

• Since most long-lasting lip colors provide a matte finish, if you prefer a glossier look, add a touch of clear gloss over them. Used alone, lip glosses are the least long-lasting lip colors.

• Try not to lick your lips. It takes the lipstick off.

• Although lip liners are not meant to color your whole lip, I use liner to do just that—cover my lips; it lasts longer than lipstick. Most women find their lips hold the color better when they use liner than when they don't.

• Don't forget that petroleum jelly adds gloss and also heals chapped lips. It's also a good base for the lip colors you mix yourself.

Lip Colors and Dyes

In the past several years a number of pigments have been tested by the National Cancer Institute because of concern from the U.S. Food and Drug Administration. Several have been found to be cancer causing (carcinogenic). The carcinogens include: D & C (Drug and Cosmetic) reds numbers 19, 37, 8, and 9, and these have been banned. The safe dyes tested include: D & C red numbers 21 and 27, and D & C orange number 5. Laws require that packages state which dyes have been used in products. I can't stress this enough: read your labels!

• BLUSHER •

If you need an instant healthy glow, pinch your cheeks. It's the quickest, easiest, cheapest blusher. I do it every time I step in front of a TV camera.

A blush can give you a glow and balance the color of your eyes and lips. That's why many women put their eye makeup on first, then a light blush, and then lip color. After you apply lip color, decide if you need more blusher. It all must balance out.

Blushers can be cream, gel, or powder. The type you select depends on your skin type and the time of day. You can use a brighter blush at night.

Some women don't like gel because they say it stains the skin. Women with oily skin often prefer gels because they think cream blushers make their skin oilier. Others prefer lip gloss or lipstick over regular blusher.

I've made a good blusher by mixing lipstick or gloss in the palm of my hand with a little petroleum jelly or hand lotion. I've also used lip gloss alone to get the "school girl" glow of some famous actresses. I rub lip gloss (or cream blush) into my fingers, dab in three or four places for a "blush of nature," and then rub gently to smooth it out.

I like to mix up my own blusher shades. Did you ever think about mixing your own shades with powdered blusher, or blending cream and gel blusher? One morning, in my bathroom lab, I experimented with six different bits of powdered blusher colors and made a great new shade.

Because I like to wear gel blusher in the morning and afternoon for its natural look, I decided to mix up all the bits of powdered blush together and add them to a dab of petroleum jelly in my palm. I worked the powdered blush into the jelly with my nail file, mixed it well, and then tested a little of my new blusher shade on the inside of my wrist—where the skin is usually most like facial skin.

It worked so well that I made up several little pots of my own blusher in colors that I like to wear—lighter, pinker, or orange-toned shades for daytime, and deeper, red, or red-burgundy colors for night. The plus of my homemade blusher is that petroleum jelly is also one of the best skin sealers ever, keeping moisture in without irritating my skin.

When I really want my blush look to be long-lasting, I do the following, which I learned from makeup artists at TV studios: I blend the cream blush application with a small sponge; then apply powder blush of the same color, to set it just like translucent powder sets foundation. Naturally, I use a separate brush for the powdered blush application. You can get extra mileage from your blusher by lightly dusting translucent powder over the powdered blush as a finishing touch to your makeup.

Applying Blusher

Most cosmetologists agree that the best place for cheek color is where it would naturally be on your face. After you've done some exercise or after that tennis game, check your mirror to see where your natural blush is. If the sun were to give you a blush it would be on the tops of your cheekbones, so find your cheekbones by sucking in your cheeks or just feeling for them with your fingers.

Apply and blend blush along the line from the center of your cheekbone and out toward your temples. Most women find that placing dots of blusher along the cheekbone and blending them with their fingers or, better yet, a moist sponge, is a good way to get a natural look. Powdered blushers are usually applied and blended with a sable brush.

Apply blusher according to the shape of your face:

• *Oval Face:* put rounds of color on the "apples" of your cheeks, right below the centers of your eyes; blend color out along your cheekbones toward the corners of your eyes.

• *Round Face:* put inverted triangles of color on top of cheekbones, under the outer two-thirds of your eyes; blend up and out toward eye corners and ears.

• *Long or Narrow Face:* put rectangular line of color along tops of cheekbones, under the outer third of eyes, and all the way out to the ear. Blend up along hairline a little past the eyebrow lines.

• *Square Face:* apply triangles of color so that the widest parts are below cheekbones and the points are beneath the center of each eye. Blend sharply up and toward hairline.

The Right Light

Since office lights glare down on you from above, you'll look healthier under them if you use a little blush on your forehead. Just use a little blush; you don't want to look too made up at work.

In the evening, artificial lights wash out color, so you need to use stronger shades and more blusher to look good. You can get a little extra color at night by applying a halo of lightly brushed blusher all around your face, blending it well. For an all-over glow, don't forget to brush some blusher or dab some rouge lightly across your earlobes, elbows, cleavage, and on your heels when you are wearing sandals.

What Kind of Blush Do You Wear Where?

Some experts recommend cream blusher for day because they say powders can look grainy in natural light. Shiny creams and gels tend to look somewhat oily under artificial light.

Many cosmeticians say that cream blush works better for normal or dry skin and powder blush is best for oily or blemished skin.

If cream blushers make your skin break out, here's how you can get a more translucent glow of cream blush from a powdered blusher. Powder your face with translucent powder; then apply powdered blusher in layers, a little at a time. When you have enough color, take a slightly damp makeup sponge and press it lightly over the area to soak up all the excess powder.

Blusher Colors

The general rule is that fair skin with pink overtones or "cool-toned" skin is flattered by pink to purple shades of blusher; and yellow or olive "warm-toned" skin looks best if brownish, peach, or taupe blushers are used.

A blusher that's a bit darker than your skin's natural color will brighten your skin. The darker your skin, the more intense color you can put on your cheeks. Peach tones warm pale skin. Clear red is a color for most skin tones.

Powder blushers blend well with natural skin tones, but remember that the same powder blusher shades do not look the same on all skins.

Your best bet is to experiment when you aren't going anywhere and can color your skin the same way you used to use crayon in your coloring books.

Some women don't like to wear foundation makeup at all. They get facial color by applying transparent bronze or clear pinky-beige shades of blusher. Try different shades from samples at cosmetic counters.

No matter what color or type of blusher you prefer, it's best to apply it a little at a time. It is easier to add more than it is to remove an overly generous application. Taking it off sometimes leaves the rest of your makeup looking blotchy. When you are accenting your eyes you'll probably want to wear less blusher—heavy makeup on both eyes and cheeks looks too made up. If you use strong lip color, you will need a strong shade of blusher. Stronger colors are also needed under artificial evening lights, when you generally use a heavier hand with your makeup.

• *SUBSTITUTES: MAKEUP MONEY SAVERS* •

Who says you shouldn't accept substitutes? Here are some of my favorites:

• *Applicators:* cotton swabs help blend eye makeup and dab at flecks you want to remove. Dip them into your economy-size bottle of mineral oil. Dipped in nail polish remover, swabs help you clean up your mistakes along the edges of your nails. They push back cuticles when you manicure. They get excess makeup out of crevices near your eyes, nose, and mouth. If you need a swab, and don't have a commercially made one, wet a wooden toothpick, orangewood stick, or end of a shadow brush, and wrap it with cotton; twirl to firmness with your fingers, making certain that the point of the toothpick is well padded. Wetting the end helps the cotton stick.

• *Bath Powder:* to get the most out of the expensive stuff, mix a box of expensive bath powder with an equal amount of baby powder, cornstarch, or baking soda. (This can also be a good, inexpensive, homemade deodorant.)

• *Blusher:* lipstick or lipstick mixed with petroleum jelly or with liquid foundation can color cheeks rosy.

• *Cold Cream:* all-vegetable shortening, petroleum jelly, mineral oil, or baby oil will substitute for commercial products.

• *Face Powder:* baby powder works as well as store-bought powders. Just puff or brush on lightly and buff off excess. You can set it with a damp sponge, just like regular powder. Cornstarch is another substitute for face powder; use it like baby powder.

• *Lip Gloss:* did you know that one of the reasons girls in beauty contests can smile so much is that they have a secret helper? Performers of all sorts like to put petroleum jelly on their lips and *inside* their lips to keep them moist. Anyone who has to speak before the public, even if it's only to your neighborhood PTA, can get rid of that "cotton mouth" feeling by using petroleum jelly this way. I guarantee it—you'll never smile as well without it once you get used to using it.

• *Pumice Stone:* try nylon net or an emery board instead.

• *Sachet:* toss your old body powder puff into drawers or closets that need freshening.

• *Sponge:* make your own wedged-shaped makeup sponges for dabbing on, blending, and setting makeup by cutting up a cheap, one-inch-thick kitchen sponge. The fine-holed foamy sponges work best, but any sponge will do. Just mark off rectangles on your sponge that are one inch wide by two inches long, or whatever size you prefer. Next, make a diagonal line from opposite corners of the rectangles—an N—cut, and there you have a whole bunch of cheap makeup wedges that will go into the corners and crevices of your face. Let's hope there aren't too many of those, hm? The wedges also are useful to stick between your toes when you polish your toenails.

Chapter 9

ALL ABOUT FRAGRANCE

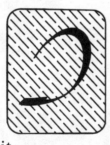sn't it nice to enjoy your favorite perfume? I always make sure to apply it to my wrists so that I can get a fragrance fix whenever I feel like it.

Many women have trouble picking a scent that blends with their own body chemistry. Even if you find the perfect scent and use it for many years, did you know that your body chemistry can change due to your taking new medications, such as birth control pills and for other reasons too? A change in body chemistry can change whatever scent you're wearing.

Another problem is that, if you have been wearing the same scent for many years, you get so used to it you don't actually smell it anymore. (This has happened to me.) You're apt to unknowingly put too much on. (You know what I mean—haven't you walked past people and practically fainted dead away from the overpowering scent?) Some people call this nose fatigue. Whatever it is, we all need to be more aware of it.

A good rule of thumb (or nose) is if, thirty minutes after you've applied a fragrance, you can still smell the scent without actually taking a sniff of your skin, you have probably overdone it.

• *SOME COMMON SCENTS* •

• *Essence:* these are the fixatives and pure oils, natural or synthetic (most are synthetic), that provide the scent. Expensive essences can contain as many as two thousand different oils and fixatives blended together.

• *Oils:* these come from flowers, roots, and plants; some are synthetic. Did you know that it takes about four thousand pounds—that's two tons—of rose petals to get just one pound of rose oil?

• *Fixatives:* these come from animals, resins, and mosses; many are synthetic. For example, ambergris, the fatty substance taken from whales, is now manufactured synthetically. Fixatives hold the fragrance components together.

• *Alcohol:* this is used to dilute and carry the smell and radiate it as the alcohol evaporates. Grain alcohol is usually used. Some people like to get one more turn from the very last of expensive fragrance by adding a dab of alcohol or vodka to the empty bottle to "rinse" it out.

• *Perfume:* this is about 70 to 85 percent alcohol (usually grain alcohol) and 15 to 30 percent essence. Different fragrances vary in percentages.

• *Toilet Water:* the strength between perfume and cologne is called toilet water.

• *Cologne:* this is about 88 to 95 percent alcohol and 5 to 12 percent essence.

• *PICKING THE RIGHT SCENT FOR YOU* •

When you shop for perfume, don't test more than two or three scents at a time. Otherwise, you'll develop nose fatigue and probably won't be able to distinguish one scent from another. Actually, it's best to try just two, one on each wrist; then sample two more the next time you're shopping. Make a third test of the two "winners" of the first two tests, and you'll probably be happy with your choice.

When shopping for perfume, try taking along some pill bottles containing cotton balls; use the sample sprays at the perfume counter on the cotton balls; then take the scents home to test later. This way, you can make a better judgment of what you like.

Cleansing Your Sniffer

Sometimes, smelling the sulfur in a match head as it burns and is blown out will help cleanse your "smeller" between sniff tests of a fragrance. Unfortunately, most department stores don't appreciate you lighting matches at their perfume counter.

Buying Your Favorite

If you think you've found the scent you like, buy it in its cheapest form—as a sachet, talc, lotion, or after-bath splash. Then you can test it for long-range use before buying the expensive perfume. I know many women who dab on bath oil the way you'd dab on perfume—it's cheaper and long-lasting too.

Tell everyone what your favorite scent is, so you don't end up receiving bottles of perfume you don't like. How many of us have untouched bottles of fragrance sitting on our bathroom shelves that smelled good on the salesperson who waited on our husbands or boyfriends?

You can use up the fragrances you just can't wear by scenting linen closets (put some on a sponge or cotton ball and place it in the closet), or other places that need help. And if you haven't liked a scent in the past, try again; sometimes your mood affects your reaction to a scent; or your body chemistry could have changed so it will work for you even if it didn't before.

A System for Scent Selection

Here's an interesting way to pick the right scent—for you or for someone else—that I learned from Jerry Ebeier, a perfumer in San Antonio. He claims a 97 percent accuracy rate in perfume selection with this method of matching fragrances to eye colors.

• Brown-eyed people can wear heavy or spicy fragrances such as Chloe, because they tend to tone down a fragrance.
• Blue-eyed people need lighter scents, such as L'Air du Temps, because they can't tone down a fragrance.

• Green-eyed people are the in-betweeners. Some of them can use heavy fragrances, but most prefer lighter fragrances.
• Gray-eyed people usually use a very light fragrance.

Some fragrances are dual fragrances and suit those who wear light scents as well as those who opt for heavy, spicy scents. Dual fragrances are usually the best-sellers.

Seasons affect your choice of scent, too. Lighter fragrances are good in warmer weather; heavier in colder weather.

• *WEARING YOUR FRAGRANCE* •

You probably will want to wear the lighter versions of your fragrance in the daytime—splash, toilet water, cologne—and add perfume, which is heavier, at night. But don't try to wear different scents at the same time; you'll be back to having people swoon as you pass by. Matching your perfume, cologne, talc, and other fragrance accessories is usually better than a mix of strange scents.

Shop alone for scents so you don't end up with something that, because of individual body chemistry, smells good on your shopping companion and not so good on you.

If, after all the testing, you still can't find the right scent, try the men's department. There's no rule that says women can't wear men's cologne, and a light aftershave splash may be just what you were looking for in a summer freshener!

• *SCENTING YOURSELF* •

We all have our own favorite tips for using fragrances. Here are some of mine:

• Fragrances put on damp skin seem to keep their fragrance longer.
• Some experts say that perfume applied with an atomizer clings to your skin better.
• Apply perfume to your "pulse points"—backs of knees, crooks of the elbows, wrists, cleavage, and behind your ears.
• Spray cologne on tired feet, even over your hose. It feels so

good, especially when you're traveling and have been trudging all over who knows where!

• *Don't* wear perfume before sunning yourself; it can cause a photosynthetic reaction on your skin—brown blotches or rashes. Instead, scent something you're carrying along with you (not your towel, because if you did you'd be wiping perfume on yourself every time you dried off).

• Some women, especially those with dry skin, like to put a dab of petroleum jelly on their skin before applying perfume; they say the petroleum jelly, like oil, helps hold the scent on longer.

• I know many women who like to spray fragrance on the hems of their clothing. But beware: the alcohol in the product could harm the fabric, as could any of the other ingredients. Actually, fragrances are made to work with your body chemistry, so spraying your clothing may just be a waste.

• *Keep* your fragrance away from jewelry—it can damage pearls and some other soft stones.

• *SAVING SCENTS* •

Fragrances aren't made to last forever, so don't collect them. The more alcohol in the product, the shorter its shelf life. Most experts say that even the strongest perfumes have a shelf life of only twelve to fourteen months. Colognes will be at their best for only six months.

Your fragrance will last longer if you store it in a cool place. Some people like to stash it in the fridge—cool cologne is a summertime favorite. Do *not* store a fragrance on a sunny window shelf. Heat makes fragrance evaporate.

Body oils react with fragrances, so avoid contaminating large bottles of fragrances. Many women save small sample bottles of their favorite fragrance and transfer small amounts from the larger container to the smaller one. Use a clean medicine dropper to transfer fragrance from one container to another, and *never* put fragrance into plastic containers; glass only! Why? Plastic alters the balance of the ingredients.

If you lose the stopper for your perfume bottle, try a pencil eraser.

Chapter 10

SHAPING UP: EXERCISE AND DIET

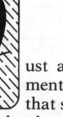

ust about everyone has some "commandments of health and beauty." Here are eight that show up on most lists:

1. Drink six to eight glasses of water daily. This advice has been around forever, it seems, but it's still good. And it won't be a chore if you just drink one glass of water with each meal (some diets tell you to drink a glass before meals to get a full feeling); drink another before your bedtime; and substitute a glass of water for a couple of your coffee breaks.

Water moisturizes your skin from within. It also dilutes the salt and minerals in your body and helps the kidneys flush them out. Drinking plenty of water can prevent kidney stones as you get older, and we've all heard terrible stories about the pain of kidney stones, which some people say makes childbirth seem like a picnic. Because it helps flush bacteria from the urinary tract, water also helps prevent urinary tract infections.

2. Find some time every day to relax. Whether you do yoga and/ or meditate, or just sit quietly by yourself, you will, by getting rid of tension, help your body avoid stress-related diseases, such as high blood pressure, ulcers, colitis, and even job burnout and sexual dysfunction. Your body needs at least twenty minutes every day to unwind, and you deserve to take the time, no matter how busy you are, because in the end it will help you be more productive. Later on in this chapter, I will give you my yoga routine, which keeps me feeling alert and energetic, no matter how hectic my schedule.

3. Start a fitness program that will strengthen your abdominal muscles. A flat tummy is attractive and makes your clothes fit better, but that's not the only plus. Most lower-back pain and other back complaints are the result of flabby abdominal muscles. Those muscles are your best "girdle"; when they give up, your weight shifts to your back muscles, which are not designed to support it, and your pelvis tilts, putting your posture out of line.

4. Do some sort of aerobic exercise daily, or at least every other day, even if it is as simple as a brisk walk.

You need at least twenty minutes of aerobic exercise done at least three times weekly to maintain proper cardiovascular conditioning. You'll find that those twenty minutes of prevention invested for your future health will also make you feel pretty good right now.

Vigorous exercise aids blood circulation, so it can help prevent varicose veins; it also helps prevent osteoporosis, which accounts for most bone fractures in postmenopausal women; it increases your metabolic rate so that you burn more calories and can keep your weight down; and it can be a factor in preventing heart disease by increasing the HDL (good) cholesterol in your blood.

Whatever exercise you choose, it should be one you enjoy, because if you don't like it, you probably won't do it. Try planning walks or other aerobic exercise with a friend so you won't be tempted to quit—but don't run or walk to the nearest ice cream store!

5. Weigh yourself often, so those pounds won't creep up on you. I like to weigh myself daily; some people prefer to do it every other day, some weekly. Doing it regularly is the key.

6. Avoid fats in your diet. A low-fat diet may prevent atherosclerosis (the buildup of plaque in the arteries) and therefore may help prevent senility, heart attacks, strokes, and high blood pressure. Studies show that women who eat low-fat diets don't have as much breast and colon cancer as those who eat fatty diets.

7. Be sure to get enough calcium—in low-fat yogurt, skim milk, cheese, sardines, salmon, and dark green vegetables—to prevent osteoporosis after menopause.

8. Include fiber (roughage) in your diet daily. You'll find it in whole-grain cereals, salad greens, fresh fruits, such as unpeeled apples and pears. By helping regulate your bowel habits, fiber prevents hemorrhoids and varicose veins, keeps your weight and cholesterol levels down, and, according to recent studies, may prevent colon cancer.

• *DIET—IS IT A DIRTY WORD?* •

I think Richard Simmons is right when he says *diet* is a dirty word. I don't think of myself as being on a diet; I just think about watching what I eat. Sometimes, I have to admit, I watch myself eat a lot, and sometimes I watch myself not eat a lot. I'll bet you do the same thing.

My main secret is that I drink a lot of liquids. I make a point of drinking six to eight glasses of water a day, and this is in addition to the tea, diet sodas, etc. that I seem to inhale.

I start off the day with a glass of water; I have another at midmorning when I start thinking about lunch, one big glass of water before lunch, the same in midafternoon and after work, and then one before the evening meal. Also, if I feel hungry after dinner or get up in the middle of the night for a snack, my snack is water.

When I was in college, I was infamous for getting up in the middle of the night for a snack, and my friends could always find me at the candy machine between 2:00 and 4:00 A.M. When I had an attack of the munchies, I could actually stumble in my sleep down to the candy machine and back. Now, I drink a glass of water while I read for a few minutes in bed before I go back to sleep. Believe me, if you drink a glass of water—and that's room temperature, not with ice, which is for sipping—your little tummy will have a head start on being filled up so that when you get around to eating, you will be less apt to gorge and eat more than you really need to.

But what I do may not be for everybody. Some experts believe that folks who retain fluids, especially if a lot of salt is in the meal, shouldn't drink too much water before meals. But they encourage those who do not retain fluids to drink water.

There is a difference between what I call "stomach hungry" and "tongue hungry." Is it your tummy that is saying, "I'm hungry, feed me," or is it your tongue that is saying, "Gee, that would taste good"? You know you really aren't hungry, but the noon whistle blows and it's supposed to be lunchtime, so like Pavlov's dogs, you begin to think you're hungry; or you walk past a bakery, and your nose goes into overdrive, making your tongue send those green lights to your brain to tell your feet, "Stop, go back for a cheese danish." So you do, knowing that your stomach doesn't need food. Officially, this is called an "oral fixation" or "an emotional need for a type of food" or "the need to chew." I think "tongue hungry" says it!

There are people who associate certain types of food with certain emotions—for example, chewing when angry. If you are one of them, recognizing that you have the problem is the first step toward solving it.

My worst temptations to eat or nibble come when I'm with people who are doing the same. I call it the animal herd instinct—you eat because the herd is eating. Here's how I cope with my herd instincts. I play a game with myself; I repeat over and over, "No, I am really not hungry. Yes, it would taste good, but the taste is going to last only a few seconds, or just a minute or two, and is that worth what is going to happen to my waist, hips, and thighs?"

Often, I deal with herd eating the way I deal with finding something on sale when I'm not really sure that I want or need the item. I think about it for five or ten minutes, then if the urge is still there, I go ahead and eat (or buy). Many times, just going through the mental process of thinking about eating a piece of chocolate pecan pie, bite for bite, is enough. Remember the old saying, anticipation is greater than realization? Well, I think that applies to fattening foods, too.

My snack controls may sound silly to some people, but, believe me, they have saved me from devouring an entire bag of cookies or a half of a chocolate peanut butter cake in one sitting. Have you ever ended up eating a half of a cake when all you were trying to do is take a small slice off each end to make the cut edge even? It's easy to do; first a little slice here, a second slice there, and pretty soon half the cake is gone before you've evened it up. Better put a cake cover over the whole thing so that you can't see it. In fact, cover up all food temptations, and keep foods in opaque containers to avoid having to look at them.

Just about everyone who has lost any amount of weight has diet advice for other dieters. Some of the advice is good; but some of it can cause serious health problems. When I want to lose a few pounds, I eat lots of vegetables, both raw and stir fried. When I'm eating out, I ask the waiter to serve the salad dressing (with all those extra fats in the oil) on the side, or I have none at all. I don't like my salad to drown in dressing anyway. When I order fish, I look for fish that is poached in wine, instead of smothered with heavy sauce. Often, even broiled fish and meats have been brushed with so much fat that they aren't low-cal anymore. When I am eating out, I ask how the food is prepared, and then, if fat is brushed on broiled entrées, I ask to have mine without fat. At home, I use the recipes and calorie-cutting hints you'll find later in this chapter.

Do all the diets you read about sometimes confuse you so much that you feel as if you are driven to eat? Dietitians, the AMA (American Medical Association), and the American Heart Association warn us about fad diets, starvation diets, fasts, and other weight-loss methods that have not been properly tested—that means scientifically tested—or that have been proven to be health hazards. There are no magic diets, the AMA says. And doctors and dietitians tell us that cutting calories, getting more exercise to burn up calories, and behavior modification are the best fat fighters and weight-loss maintainers.

Here's the straight scoop from a survey of very low-calorie (fewer than one thousand calories daily) weight-reduction diets, published in the Archives of Internal Medicine and copyrighted by the AMA (American Medical Association), which divides the various fad diets into novelty diets, total fasts, protein-sparing modified fasts, and formula diets.

Novelty Diets

Emphasis is on eating certain foods that are said to have magical properties that make you lose weight, such as grapefruit, pumpkins and carrots, or steak and tomatoes. The "magic" is in certain foods that are supposed to oxidize body fat, cut appetite, remove toxins, or increase your metabolism. What really happens is that you lose weight because you are cutting calories as you eat the recommended foods, or the limited food choices get so boring that you lose your appetite and eat less. Some novelty diets require use of certain substances, such as kelp, lecithin, and apple-cider vinegar, which are supposed to decrease appetite or change your metabolism so that food energy is not absorbed by your body or at least not deposited as fat in your body.

The problem with novelty diets, the AMA says, is that they don't teach dieters how to maintain a weight loss, some of them are so nutritionally unbalanced that they are hazardous to health, and some may cause chronic health problems. According to the report, the Beverly Hills diet may even foster eating habits that lead to weight gain.

Some novelty diets studied by the AMA are: the rice diet, the Beverly Hills diet, the K-28 diet, the Zen macrobiotic diet.

Total Fasting

The U.S. Public Health Service warns that total fasting should never be attempted without medical supervision. Fasting leads to ketosis and the wasting of muscle tissue. It causes extreme chemical imbalances in the body and has caused irregular heartbeats in people with cardiovascular disease when they exercised after fasting. Headaches, nausea, and weakness are among the side effects of fasting. And studies show that weight lost by total fasting rarely stays off.

PSMF (Protein-Sparing Modified Fast)

A semistarvation fast with a very low-calorie, high-protein diet, this is now under investigation. Dangerous for pregnant women, children, adolescents, patients with kidney or liver disease, anyone with heart disease, and certain diabetics, the PSMF can lead to reduced tolerance to the cold, brittle nails, hair loss, and dry skin, as well as postural dizziness in some patients.

Formula Diets

Designed to be alternatives to total fasting, these involve formulas that are supposed to provide adequate nutrition without calorie counting. But the AMA survey says that no formula diet absolutely fulfills the nutritional requirements of everyone, and formula dieting does not teach obese people new eating habits for keeping those pounds off. Lack of fiber is a concern (some formulas are now adding fiber), along with the chemical imbalances caused in the bodies of formula dieters. Postural dizziness, dehydration, vomiting, diarrhea, constipation, irregular heartbeats, and other symptoms have been reported. Formula diets have led to some deaths.

Among the formula diets surveyed by the AMA were the Cambridge diet, the last-chance diet, defined formula and mini-cal diets.

The conclusion of the AMA study was that an obese patient on a diet of fewer than one thousand calories needs vitamin supplements, possibly the addition of a formula diet, and supervision. The goal is to lose weight, keep it off, and improve health with a diet that suits the patient's life-style. The most important part of any weight-loss program is a weight-maintenance plan, the AMA survey concludes. The survey was conducted by Stephen R. Newmark, M.D., and Beverly Willamson, M.S., R.D. (R.D. stands for registered dietitian, a dietitian who is certified in this particular field. Many "nutritionists" give diet advice, but are not qualified or trained to be registered dietitians. Some are actually self-taught, and certificates should be investigated before you get involved in a health program.)

At the time this book was being researched, the top ten diets were rated by Dr. Paul LaChance and registered dietitian Michele C. Fisher of Rutgers University. The diets rated were: Beverly Hills, F-Plan, Pritikin 1,200, Pritikin 700, I Love America, Richard Simmons, I Love New York, Scarsdale, Atkins, and Stillman.

Two weeks of the ten diets' menu plans were studied, and none met the U.S. Recommended Daily Allowance for all thirteen vitamins and minerals. Some were short in B vitamins, calcium, and iron and zinc. Nearly all called for more protein than necessary, and several were too high in cholesterol and sodium, but too low in fiber. According to these experts, ideal diets contain two-thirds of foods from plant sources (cereal, grain, beans, vegetables, fruits) and one-third from animal sources (meat, dairy). Most American diets are 60 percent animal and 40 percent vegetable.

The F-Plan diet, a high-fiber diet from England, is the best provider of nutrients, and the I Love New York and Pritikin 1,200 diets provide at least half of the vitamins and minerals needed. Diets providing the least amount of vitamins and minerals were Scarsdale, Richard Simmons, Beverly Hills, Stillman, and Atkins.

• *LOSING WEIGHT* •

In any diet, the weight that you lose at first is mostly due to loss of water; if you stick to your reduced-calorie diet, you should stabilize at losing one or two pounds weekly. Since each pound of body fat equals 3,500 calories, to lose two pounds weekly, you need to cut 7,000 calories from your week's intake of food, or 1,000 calories a day. Exercise, such as tennis, burns up only 350 calories per hour when played strenuously, so you still have to cut your food intake even if you exercise to tone up and increase your metabolism.

• *FIGURING OUT CALORIE NEEDS* •

A moderately active adult woman older than twenty-two can use this simple rule for figuring out calorie needs: multiply desired weight by 15 calories per pound. For example, if your desired weight is 120 pounds, $120 \times 15 = 1,800$; so that means you need 1,800 calories per day to maintain your 120-pound weight. To lose any weight, you need to decrease your calories by 500 calories per day for a one-pound weekly weight loss or 1,000 calories per day for a two-pound weekly weight loss by diet and/or exercise.

It can't be said often enough—a slow, steady weight loss of one or two pounds per week is best for your health. And weight lost slowly is more likely to stay off.

• *BALANCING YOUR DIET* •

Sometimes it seems like balancing a diet is more strenuous exercise than jogging, but if you think about the "whys" of food, it's easy to think about balance. We eat to get energy, to build and repair tissue, and to regulate our body functions. That's why we need to get carbohydrates, proteins, fats, vitamins, minerals, and water each day.

Carbohydrates

They give us energy better than any other part of our diet and are the cheapest and least caloric (half the calories per ounce of fats) component of our diet. We need about 50 percent carbohydrates in our diets.

Protein

Protein is the substance from which body tissues are made, and so it's needed for growth and repair; it's also needed to make body chemicals, such as enzymes and hormones. Many people think protein is the most important diet component. Well, they're wrong. Generally, Americans eat too much protein. We actually only need 15 to 20 percent protein of our total calorie intake.

Fats

We can't eliminate all fats from our diet because fats are the most concentrated source of energy, and because they are digested and used more slowly by the body, they keep hunger pangs away longer. Fats have more than two times the calories of protein or carbohydrates and should be eaten in moderation, making up about 30 percent of our diet.

Vitamins and Minerals

Vitamins and minerals regulate our body's functions and most experts agree that people who eat a variety of foods in a well-balanced diet get enough vitamins and minerals. Women need twice the iron as men need and should include liver, eggs, nuts, leafy green vegetables, raisins, and enriched breads in their diets to prevent iron deficiency and the resulting fatigue, loss of endurance and strength, and inability to concentrate. Lack of calcium between ages twenty and forty contributes to osteoporosis in old age.

Water

We need water to produce energy, for endurance, for elimination of body waste, and for body-temperature control, especially when we exercise strenuously.

• CHOOSING FOODS FOR NUTRITION •

We have all heard of the five basic food groups from our mothers, doctors, and health classes at one time or another. And no matter how many different kinds of diets people go on, in the end, the most helpful are those that get us to eat from those five basic food groups as a lifetime eating plan. So here we go again with the five basic food groups:

Meat/Poultry/Fish/Beans Group

This food group also includes eggs, nuts, and seeds. We need two servings daily to get the protein, phosphorous, magnesium, zinc, iron, and other minerals and vitamins contained in this group. It's best to vary our selections from this group.

Buy lean cuts of meat with minimum marbling (fat layers), and remember that all meat fat is saturated fat, the fat you want to avoid. Poultry contains less saturated fat than beef, pork, or veal, and you can get rid of even more fat by removing the skin from chicken or turkey before cooking. Avoid duck and goose, which are high in fat. Game, such as venison, rabbit, dove, quail, and squirrel, are lower in fat. Fish fat is polyunsaturated and contains less fat than other "meats," unless you insist on frying it. It has fewer calories, too. Shellfish are included in the fish category; but in low-cholesterol diets, shrimp and crayfish are not included. They are high in cholesterol (one six-ounce serving of shrimp equals one egg yolk in cholesterol).

Meat substitutes are cottage and other cheeses, peas, beans, and other vegetable proteins.

Milk/Cheese Group

Adult women need two servings from this group to get calcium, riboflavin, protein, and vitamins. Teens and pregnant or nursing women need more. The milk/cheese group includes yogurt, ice cream, ice milk, cottage and other cheeses and can substitute for meat servings.

When you are on a low-fat diet look for skim dairy products, which contain less than 1 percent butterfat. Low-fat products contain 1 to 2 percent butterfat, and high-fat dairy products contain as much as 80 percent butterfat. Most hard cheeses contain a lot of saturated fat. Among the cheeses with 30 or more percent fat are Jarlsberg (45), cream (33), cheddar (31), camembert, colby, hoop (30-plus).

Bread/Cereal Group

You need four servings of breads, cereals, pasta, baked goods, and rice (not each, four total) to get the B vitamins, iron, and fiber your body requires. Bread/cereal foods should be enriched or fortified or made from whole grains. These foods supply energy. Pastas, low-fat crackers, starchy vegetables, commercially prepared soups, and alcohol all contain carbohydrates, but the complex carbohydrates —breads, cereals, pastas, low-fat crackers, and starchy vegetables —are better food choices than baked goods or alcohol because they also supply vitamins and minerals.

Commercial baking mixes and other convenience foods usually use saturated fats, so if you are on a low-cholesterol diet, avoid packaged foods or commercial mixes.

Fruit/Vegetable Group

You need four servings from this group daily to provide vitamins in your diet, and this should include a vitamin C source, such as citrus fruits, melons, berries, or tomatoes, and a vitamin A source, such as deep yellow or dark green vegetables. Also add unpeeled fruits and vegetables and those with edible seeds, such as berries, for fiber. No fruits and vegetables contain cholesterol, and nearly all are low-fat.

Fruits and vegetables are low in calories and will stay that way as long as you don't season them with butter, bacon fat, salt pork, or ham hocks. Try other herbs and spices if you don't like your veggies plain, but even if you're not used to it, try plain veggies once in a while. You'd be surprised how good vegetables are when they aren't smothered in fats and rich sauces.

Also remember that dried beans and peas are economical, low-cholesterol substitutes for meat. Check labels of frozen and canned fruits and vegetables for sugar and salt content. Many diets allow unlimited amounts of raw or cooked dark green or yellow vegetables such as lettuce, celery, and carrots because they are good filler-uppers when you are cutting back on calories. Whole-grain bread is also a filler-upper when you are cutting down.

Fats and Sweets Group

You can include this group if you can afford the calories. Butter, margarine, mayonnaise and other fats, oils, candy, jams, jellies, syrups, and other sweets belong to this group.

Since a high-cholesterol level in your blood is associated with heart disease and atherosclerosis, you need to avoid saturated fats, which increase cholesterol levels, and eat polyunsaturated fats, which reduce blood cholesterol.

Saturated fats are usually solid at room temperature and are found in animal-origin foods such as cream, whole milk, and cheeses made from whole milk,

Coconut, coconut oil, and palm kernel oil are vegetable sources of saturated fats, and these fats are most often found in nondairy coffee creamers, nondairy whipped toppings, nondairy sour creams, cake mixes, and other commercial baked products.

Chocolate is also vegetable-origin saturated fat, but cocoa powder and carob powder have the fat removed. So unlike chocolate chips, semisweet baking chocolate, German chocolate, and chocolate candy, cocoa and carob powder have no saturated fats.

Polyunsaturated fats are liquid at room temperature, and include safflower, corn, soybean, and cottonseed oils. Fish fat is also polyunsaturated. All oils contain the same amount of calories, but since safflower oil is the most polyunsaturated oil, and lowers cholesterol most in the body, half as much safflower oil produces the same cholesterol-lowering effect in the body as any other oil.

Monounsaturated fats, such as olive oil, peanut oil, olives, peanuts, avocados, and peanut butter, are considered "neutral" fats because they neither raise nor lower cholesterol levels in the body. They contain the same amount of calories as the other fats and oils, but are not recommended for people on low cholesterol diets because they do not lower cholesterol levels.

• SHOPPING FOR FOOD •

Even the most knowledgeable of us get confused when we try to read food labels for nutrition information or because we are trying to avoid eating some additive or fats and salt.

For example, "natural" doesn't have a legal definition or standard, so when you think you are getting something naturally pure, safe, or nutritious, you can be getting anything. A "natural-flavored" chocolate cookie could have natural chocolate flavor but artificial color, as well as other ingredients you want to avoid. "Naturally sweetened" is not necessarily healthier, since honey is still sugar. If you are trying to keep sugar out of your diet, sweetening with honey instead of cane sugar isn't the way to go. And although "sugar-free" means no sugar, it can still mean the same number of calories.

"Reduced calorie" means that the food in the package has at least one-third fewer calories than similar foods in similar packages, but it is not necessarily low calorie.

Foods with labels that say they provide "food energy" don't necessarily contain any special ingredients to provide extra energy; foods contain calories and calories provide energy, so even fattening foods provide energy, as well as more calories than you need.

"Wheat bread" is not necessarily whole-wheat bread, and "no preservatives" is not necessarily healthier because foods with no preservatives or no artificial coloring can still contain fat, sugar, and salt.

Manufacturers decide how many ounces are in a serving, so when you are determining the number of calories you will get from a serving, base your figuring on the amount you eat. A label can say that a twelve-ounce can contains four servings, but remember that it then has four three-ounce servings, and if there are fifty calories per serving, it's fifty calories for three ounces. If you eat six-ounce servings, then you are eating one hundred calories.

You can find pocket-size brand-name calorie counters at supermarket magazine stands that will help you keep track when you shop and when you are eating out at chain restaurants.

Fast-Food Fat

Dieters can eat some fast-food items, but you need to know which ones fit a reducing regime. The problem with most fast foods is that they are high in fat content, plus it's so tempting to order extras like french fries, which contain about ninety-nine calories of fat per order. (Compare that to no fat in a plain baked potato!). Forty to 50 percent of the calories in most fast foods are fat, and burgers and fries are big offenders.

HOW TO CUT THE FAT FROM A FEW FAST FOODS

• Have a McDonald's English muffin without butter to save 35 calories.

• Have a Burger King Whopper without mayo to save 159 calories.

• Have a McDonald's Big Mac without sauce and save 105 calories.

• Have a Shakey's pizza without salami, olives, sausage, or pepperoni to save 23 to 52 calories.

• Have a Pizza Hut pizza without pepperoni, pork, or extra cheese for a saving of 27 to 144 calories.

• Have Original Recipe instead of Extra Crispy Kentucky Fried Chicken Dinner to save 95 calories.

• Step up to the salad bar anywhere and don't ladle on dressing to save 100 to 133 calories. Don't forget that regular cheese is about 100 calories per ounce, that croutons are sometimes butter brushed, and ham or bacon has more calories than turkey or chicken.

Fast Food as Real Food

Although most fast food is high in calories, fat, and sodium, a survey made by the American Council on Science and Health did show that a meal such as a burger and fries does provide part of the government's recommended daily nutritional needs by adding protein, iron, niacin, thiamin, riboflavin, the B vitamins, calcium, and phosphorous to your diet. In fact, for most people, a typical fast-food meal contains at least one-third of daily protein needs, and nutritional studies of junk-food snacks indicate that they aren't totally junky.

PIZZA AS A MEAL Pizza, for example, with its bread, cheese, tomatoes, peppers, and mushrooms, does represent the basic four food groups and so it's nutritious as a meal, even if the cheese and tomato sauce contain salt and the cheese contains fat. The trick is not to eat pizza, at four or five hundred calories a piece, as a snack; eat it as a meal. I order vegetarian pizza with half the normal amount of cheese and really cut calories.

ICE CREAM Did you know that ice cream has less sugar than sweetened yogurt? But don't run out and have a chocolate sundae: it does have more fat than yogurt, and depending on the fat content of individual brands, you get from 135 to 175 calories per half cup of vanilla ice cream and more calories with chocolate and other flavors. But you also get protein and calcium. You'll save about 30 calories per half cup if you substitute ice milk for ice cream.

POPCORN Without butter and salt, this good source of fiber has only 40 calories per cupful if made with oil; only 23 calories if made without oil. Substitute two cups popcorn for one-fourth cup peanuts and save 120 calories.

PEANUTS About thirty nuts will give you 115 to 120 calories, and a lot of protein. The best way to eat peanuts for nutrition and health is freshly shelled and unsalted.

CHOCOLATE BARS Even a milk chocolate bar has nutritious ingredients—calcium and some others—but an ounce and a half of milk chocolate equals more than 220 calories. If you crave chocolate and won't substitute carob powder, try around fifty small chocolate-covered raisins instead of a one-ounce piece of chocolate candy. You will save 25 calories and add the benefit of raisins' iron.

FRIES Even french fries provide potassium, B vitamins, and iron, but they are also high in salt and fat and contain 210 to 220 calories per six-ounce serving.

Less Fat, Fewer Calories, Less Sodium

Here are some general hints for eating fast foods and snacks with less fat, calories, and sodium:

• Cut fat by not ordering deep-fat fried anything and by not having cheese, mayo, ketchup, or any special sauces on your burgers.
• Cut calories by ordering a small order of fries instead of a large one, by ordering the smallest size of burger offered, and by getting diet soda or iced tea instead of a shake.
• Add more vitamins and minerals to your meal by substituting coleslaw or salad for fries, and by ordering juices or milk to drink.
• Cut down on sodium by not salting your fries and avoiding pickles, sauces, ketchup, and mustard.

• Cut out 135 calories by substituting thirty very thin three-inch pretzel sticks for thirty potato chips.

• Cut 185 calories by eating angel food or sponge cake instead of chocolate-frosted layer cake.

• Cut 75 calories per drink by making a wine spritzer of four ounces white wine, four ounces club soda, and ice instead of a mixed drink or cocktail.

• Save 50 calories by putting strained baby food fruit on your pancakes or waffles instead of two tablespoons of maple syrup. Try an old German custom: put unsweetened applesauce on pancakes —it's also less expensive than syrup. (You can also substitute mashed banana and puréed fruit for jelly on your toast to save calories.)

• Cut 60 or 65 calories by eating half an English muffin topped with one teaspoon jam instead of a sweet roll or glazed doughnut when you just have to have something sweet in the morning.

• Save 220 calories per half cup by whipping chilled evaporated skim milk instead of heavy cream.

• Cut 35 calories per slice by substituting thin for regular-sliced bread.

• Cut about 200 calories from a family meal by making your second helping vegetables, even potatoes, instead of a quarter pound of meat.

• NUTRITION THE NATURAL WAY •

I like more than 50 percent of the food I eat to be in its natural state, as is recommended by many diet experts. I prefer my vegetables raw or steamed and include high-fiber grains and lots of fresh fruits in my daily diet. I also avoid meats and eat fish and vegetable proteins, such as beans or whole grains, and eat plenty of low-fat dairy products.

Since I live in Texas, I do allow myself a good bowl of red (chili to out-of-state foreigners) about once a year. I really do believe that too much salt and too many artificial ingredients cause water-weight gain and give me puffy skin. I also think that gaining and losing weight again and again is bad for your health and appearance because it causes loss of skin tone and leaves stretch marks. That's why I try to maintain my weight with a vegetarian diet.

But before *you* decide on a vegetarian diet, you need to know how to plan your diet so that you get proper nutrition with correct protein complements. Now, that probably sounds like a lot of junk words, but all protein complementarity means is that you use the three basic combinations of foods in each meal to give your body the amino acids it needs when you don't eat meats.

Animal products are proteins with the amino acids you need; plant foods are incomplete and must be combined properly to provide amino acids. Improper planning of a vegetarian diet can result in deficiencies of protein, vitamin B-12, riboflavin, iron, calcium, zinc, magnesium, and iodine.

Protein Complements

• Grains plus legumes. Grains include products made from soy flour, cornmeal, rice, barley, whole wheat, rye, and oatmeal, such as pasta, bread, and cereal. Legumes are vegetables, such as dried beans, peas, and lentils.
• Grains plus milk products.
• Seeds, such as sesame or sunflower, plus legumes.

Kinds of Vegetarians

Generally, vegetarians eat only vegetables, fruits, grains, and nuts. They replace meat in their diets with a variety of legumes and meat substitutes, such as texturized vegetable protein, cereals, and nuts. There are three types of vegetarians:

• *Vegan:* these vegetarians do not eat any foods of animal origin at all.
• *Lactovegetarian:* these vegetarians eat dairy products but no eggs.
• *Lacto-ovo Vegetarians:* these people eat dairy products and eggs.

Vegetarian Diet Pluses

The advantages of a vegetarian diet, according to a variety of studies, are lower levels of blood fats, cholesterol, and triglycerides than meat eaters; less high blood pressure; and lower cancer risk. Vegetarian women are reported to excrete more estrogen and therefore have less of it in their blood than meat-eating women, making them less apt to get cancer. The low-fat, high-fiber diets of vegetarians along with the protection of nutrients found in vegetables, beans, and whole grains, such as vitamins A and C, are considered factors for better health and resistance to disease. (See the discussion of cancer in "Diet Facts and Fancy," later in this chapter.)

• *MY RECIPES AND CALORIE CUTTERS* •

Diet food doesn't have to taste like paste. I use diet salad dressings to perk up chicken, egg, or tuna salad, as a mixer in low-cal casseroles, and for topping on my baked potato. You've heard it before, and it's true—it's not the potato that's fattening, it's the calories that you load on it. An average potato has only one hundred calories. Here are some of my salad-dressing ideas:

Mock Italian Dressing

To low-fat yogurt, spicy mustard, or vinegar, add a few drops of water and some spices. My favorite is a bottled mix called Fancy Spices. This dressing is great for all kinds of things. If it is too tart for you, add a little artificial sweetener to cut the pucker.

Heloise's Low-fat and Cal Egg Salad

Hard-boil eggs. Use only one or two yolks, the rest egg whites (I like to chop my eggs in large pieces). Add diced water chestnuts, celery, or red cabbage for crunch, and one dill pickle. (Don't use prepared relish because it has sugar.)

Add dressing. I like to mix three to four tablespoons of low-fat yogurt, some spicy mustard, and lots of seasonings. If you are watching your salt intake, be sure to read the labels of the seasonings you add. I add hot, zingy spices such as cayenne pepper, dry hot mustard, maybe even a dash of Tabasco sauce.

You can make this salad with chicken or tuna, and you can add other bulky, crunchy, free or low-cal veggies such as celery, cabbage, carrots, and so forth. It's the dressing that saves you calories.

Sometimes I like to make egg salad scramble by mixing only one yolk and several whites. I scramble, add lots of favorite spices, mix in hot mustard, then toss with chopped lettuce and tomatoes.

When I make a vinegar-and-oil dressing, I save about thirty calories per tablespoon by going from three or four parts oil to half oil and half vinegar or lemon juice. Often, I eliminate the oil entirely and just use flavored vinegar or lemon or lime juice.

Heloise "Omeletter"

This can serve as a low-cal breakfast, lunch, or supper. Beat three to four egg whites until almost fluffy; add one egg yolk; pour into nonstick coated pan and cook over low heat. Lift edge to see if slightly brown, then, if you wish, you can put the omelette under the broiler to brown the top of it and to finish cooking it if it's a little underdone. Then add very low-cal fillings: two finely chopped olives, fresh mushrooms, shredded lettuce, sliced or chopped water chestnuts. If you like the taste of sour cream, but want to avoid calories and fat, use a tablespoon of low-fat yogurt; sprinkle with spices; enjoy.

HELOISE DIET PUMPKIN BREAD

1⅔ cup whole-wheat flour
10 to 12 packages (2 tablespoons each) artificial sweetener
1 teaspoon salt
1 to 2 teaspoons each of allspice, cinnamon, nutmeg (to overpower the artificial sweetener taste)
½ cup chopped nuts (optional—can use bran, wheat germ, sesame seeds)
2 eggs, slightly beaten
½ cup salad oil
1 cup (½ a 12-ounce can) pumpkin (can use ¾ can for a more pumpkiny taste)

Sift together dry ingredients; add nuts or seeds; mix together. Mix together eggs, oil, and pumpkin; add to dry ingredients. Pour into greased and floured loaf pans; bake at 350 degrees for 50 to 60 minutes; test for doneness with toothpick. I use two small loaf pans for this bread because then it cooks about 20 minutes faster.

Super Sippers

Here are some super sipping drinks to fill you up when you crave something and you don't exactly know what:

SPRITZER PICKER-UPPER

¾ cup grapefruit juice
¼ cup club soda

Mix, pour over ice, and enjoy, for 76 calories per serving.

PUNCHLESS PUNCH

¾ cup pineapple juice
¾ cup cranberry juice cocktail
¾ cup club soda

Mix, pour over ice. Serves two at 110 calories per 8-ounce serving.

FRUITY WHIRR

3 or 4 strawberries
Thick slice of fresh pineapple
¼ or ⅛ of fresh melon
Ice cubes

In blender, whir fruits, adding ice cubes one at a time until all is a frothy pink.

OTHER SIPPERS

Sip tea with lemon for zero calories.

Some Eight-Ounce Low-Calorie Treats

Carbonated water with a lime wedge or one tablespoon of orange juice comes to 15 calories. Sip 100 percent vegetable juice for 40 calories. Tomato juice is 50 calories. Unsweetened orange or grapefruit juice is 105 to 115 calories. Try a mix of half fruit or vegetable juice and half carbonated water to cut calories of the juice in half. Skim milk is 90 calories; 1 percent fat milk, 110 calories; 2 percent fat milk, 130 calories.

Got enough?

Just remember that most soft drinks are 100 to 125 calories per eight-ounce glass and all the calories are from sugar; juicy spritzers and milk give you nutrition instead of just sugar. Remember also that you can't load up on diet drinks if you are watching your salt intake; sodium bicarbonate—the fizz—is sodium and that's what you're trying to avoid.

PRUNE PURR LOW-CAL DESSERT

5 egg whites
1 cup prune baby food
2 tablespoons lemon juice

Beat egg whites until stiff. Fold in puréed prunes. Add lemon juice. Blend together and chill.

MARINATED MUSHROOMS

1 pound mushrooms
1 pint water
¾ cup vinegar or lemon juice
1 tablespoon polyunsaturated oil
1 pinch of thyme
1 bay leaf

Wash mushrooms. Bring water and vinegar or lemon juice to boil in saucepan; add mushrooms; cook three minutes. Add oil, thyme, and bay leaf; chill and serve. Serves 4 to 6.

GAZPACHO VERDE

2 peeled tomatoes
3 celery stalks
1 small peeled cucumber
1 small head of lettuce
1 cup orange juice
Juice of one lemon or more to taste

Combine all ingredients in a blender. Blend to combine.

Cutting Calories, Adding Nutrition

There are so many ways to cut calories and add nutrients when you are cooking at home that a whole book could be written about them. Here are just a few hints:

BREAD CRUMBS Substitute soy grits or wheat germ for bread crumbs to get extra nutrition. They will absorb liquids as well as bread in meat loaf or other recipes. You can thicken stews with rice, rice grits, buckwheat, bulgur wheat, millet, or other ground grains for extra nutrition in your gravy.

COOKIES Sandwich, chocolate chip, and shortbread cookies have more than 12 percent fat; graham crackers, ginger snaps, and fig bars have less than 12 percent fat.

PASTA TOPPERS Toss with poppy or caraway seeds and add zero calories; top with one-fourth cup meatless spaghetti sauce to add forty-five calories; top with two pats of butter or margarine to add seventy calories; use butter buds instead of butter or margarine and add only about twenty-four calories.

SANDWICH FILLERS Some sandwich innards are: turkey roll, 3 percent fat; boiled ham, 17 percent fat; bologna, 23 percent fat; cooked salami, 26 percent fat; dry salami, 38 percent fat. American cheese (pasteurized process), 25 percent fat; Swiss, 26 percent; cheddar, 33 percent; cream cheese, 35 percent fat.

Cottage cheese is only 1 percent fat, but unless it's whirred to cream-cheese consistency in a blender, it makes a weird sandwich, one that few people would find appealing.

SWEET SAVERS Use extract of brandy, rum, or others that you like to flavor desserts instead of the real liquor and/or sugar to save forty-five to sixty calories for each tablespoon of liquor eliminated.

When you make fruit pies, cut the sugar and use a third or half the amount called for in the recipe; then use extra fruit to fill the bottom crust well; don't put on a top crust at all. You'll save about eight hundred calories total on the crust alone.

If your recipe doesn't require a long, high temperature for baking and if you can add sweetener after heating, substitute nonnutritive sweetener for half the sugar. Nonnutritive sweeteners do not bake well, especially at high temperatures, although research is continuing to improve their baking capacity.

SWEET-TOOTH SNACK Raisins are as sweet as anything needs to be and the bonus is that they add iron, potassium, phosphorous, magnesium, and some B vitamins to your diet. They are 77 percent carbohydrate, just about fat free, have no cholesterol, and are low in sodium. What more could anyone ask?

When you crave sweets, sprinkle raisins over hot or cold cereal, mix them in your veggie (especially carrot) or fruit salads, put them in stuffings and sauces, or just munch a handful.

TUNA Use water-packed tuna instead of oil-packed and save 155 calories per three-and-a-half-ounce can. Water-packed tuna has 1 percent fat and oil-packed tuna has 24 percent fat. You can drain and rinse oil-packed tuna with water to help cut calories.

TURKEY Try using ground turkey in your chili and in other recipes that call for ground beef, such as meat loaf, meatballs, and casseroles; you'll make a big calorie saving if you do. Chicken or turkey, unless cooked with extra fat and sauce, are low-fat meats. White meat without skin is 2 percent fat; white meat with skin is 4 percent fat; dark meat without skin is 4 percent fat; and dark meat with skin is 6 percent fat. Beef ranges from 11 percent fat in round to 33 percent fat in a porterhouse steak. Pork ranges from 16 percent fat in the loin to 33 percent fat in spareribs.

VEGETABLE SALT Try the ground-up vegetables sold as vegetable salt if you have to restrict the salt in your diet. Even if you don't need to, you'll find good flavor with extra bits of nutrition in the table salt substitute.

VEGGIE VITAMINS Instead of peeling off some of the vitamins that you paid for when you bought your fruits and veggies, scrub instead of peel and save it all. And you'll save time, too! Also, salting vegetables before they are cooked tends to drive out nutrients; cook first and season later for best nutrition. Most important, don't cook the nutrients out of your vegetables. Stir fry in bouillon or steam, or eat them raw!

• *NUTRITION FROM A TO ZINC* •

From vitamin A to zinc, the vitamins and minerals found in your food will interact to make you healthy if you eat a well-balanced diet. There are controversies over the need for vitamin and mineral supplements. Some experts say a well-balanced diet provides all the nutrients you need, unless specific health problems or other conditions cause nutrient deficiencies. Others recommend supplements for just about everyone. Those who recommend supplements for everyone, I've noticed, are often people who *sell* them.

When you are looking for someone other than a physician to consult about your diet, you will find many people who call themselves nutritionists. Some of these nutritionists actually have legitimate certification and training, but others are self-taught or have mail-order certificates.

To determine which nutritionist to see, look for professional credentials, such as academic degrees from accredited institutions, memberships in legitimate professional organizations, such as the local American Dietetic Association (ADA) and/or a medical society, and other certifications or registrations. In addition to the ADA, other legitimate professional organizations are the American Board of Nutrition (ABN), the American Institute of Nutrition (AIN), and the American Society of Clinical Nutrition (ASCN).

A registered dietician (R.D.), such as Judy New, a good friend and a consultant on this book, is a person specially trained to use nutrition research in planning a healthy diet for you. You can find registered dietitians through physician or hospital referrals. Often registered dietitians will have their offices in medical buildings so they are conveniently located to receive physician referrals.

Vitamins

Where are they found? Which interacts with which? What do they do? What happens if you have a vitamin deficiency?

VITAMIN A (RETINOL, CAROTENE)   This is found in fish-liver oil, beef liver, apricots, broccoli, cantaloupe, carrots, eggs, sweet potatoes, dark green vegetables, yellow squash, all green and yellow fruits and vegetables, milk, butter, cheese, and yogurt.

It interacts with fats and minerals in the body.

You need it for proper use of protein, to purify the bloodstream, maintain healthy skin and tissues, prevent night blindness, protect body from bacterial and viral infections, for healthy thyroid balance. Vitamin A is thought by some to retard cancer growth. Some also say it helps delay senility and prolong life.

Deficiencies may cause acne and other skin problems, eye problems, night blindness, chronic infections.

VITAMIN B-1 (THIAMIN)   This is found in brewer's yeast, whole-grain cereals, wheat germ, milk, enriched oatmeal, brown rice, fresh pork, bran, meats and soybeans, peas, vegetables, and peanuts.

It's more effective when it interacts with other B vitamins, manganese, and vitamins C and E.

B-1 is needed to metabolize sugar and starch properly for energy, for a healthy nervous system and mental outlook. Stress increases the need for B-1 and all B-6 vitamins, some say, and B-1 is needed for growth, appetite, and the digestive tract's functions.

Deficiencies can result in cardiac muscle weakness, gastrointestinal problems, or weakness.

VITAMIN B-2 (RIBOFLAVIN)   B-2 is found in organ meats such as beef liver and tongue, fish, milk, cheese, eggs (especially the whites), beans, green leafy vegetables, plums and prunes, and nuts.

It interacts best with B-complex, B-6, niacin, and vitamin C and is water-soluble.

It aids metabolism of protein, fats, and carbohydrates; is important to good muscle tone and a healthy nervous system, skin, and eyes; works with vitamin A to maintain healthy mucous membranes in the respiratory, digestive, circulatory, and excretory tracts; aids vision, skin, nails, and hair health; and is needed in pregnancy to help the fetus's development.

Early deficiency symptoms may be sores on the eyes or in the mouth.

VITAMIN B-3 (NIACIN, NIACINAMIDE, NICOTINIC ACID, NICOTINAMIDE)   The best sources of B-3 are meat, fish, and grain products.

It interacts with other B vitamins and vitamin C.

B-3 is needed for a healthy nervous system, skin, and digestion. It helps you digest fats and absorb fat-soluble nutrients and can help you reduce the cholesterol and triglyceride levels in your body. It is also said to help prevent senility.

Deficiency is uncommon. It can result in pellagra, a disease that involves skin rashes, dementia, and diarrhea. Lack of B-3 can also cause irritability, headaches, loss of memory or appetite. Deficiency of B-3 is often found in alcoholics, diabetics, cancer patients, and those who suffer chronic diarrhea.

VITAMIN B-5 (PANTOTHENIC ACID) This is found in brewer's yeast, organ meats, egg yolk, legumes, and whole-grain cereal.

B-5 is the backbone of coenzyme. It reacts for synthesis of fatty acids, cholesterol, and sterols.

Deficiency is not easily recognized, but sometimes tenderness in heels and feet, fatigue, weakness, or leg cramps are the signs of a B-5 deficiency.

VITAMIN B-6 (PYRIDOXINE, PYRIDOXAL, PYRIDOXA-MINE) This is well distributed in plant and animal foods, such as bananas, brewer's yeast, dry kidney beans, whole-grain products, potatoes, brown rice, wheat germ, soybeans, pecans, walnuts, peanuts, green leafy vegetables, beef liver, chicken, pork, and such fish as herring, mackerel, and salmon. Heat in cooking destroys this vitamin. So does storage of some of these foods.

It interacts with other B vitamins, vitamin C, magnesium, and potassium.

B-6 is needed to metabolize protein and fat; form niacin, red blood cells, bile salts, and various hormones; prevent tooth decay by maintaining healthy teeth and facial bones; aid in normal nervous-system function; aid in chemical balance of the body fluids, regulating water excretion, energy production, and stress resistance.

Deficiencies can result in sores on the lips, tongue, or skin. If pregnant women have deficiencies in this vitamin, it can harm their babies.

VITAMIN B-12 (COBALAMIN, CYANOCOBALAMIN) This is found in lamb, pork, beef and veal liver, and kidney; such fish as salmon, sardines, herring, crab, and oysters; egg yolk; milk and other dairy products.

It interacts with other B-vitamins, vitamin C, and potassium. Taking too much vitamin C can destroy the B-12 in the food you eat.

B-12 is needed for normal functioning of body cells, especially in the bone marrow, gastrointestinal tract, and nervous system, including brain cells; it is a blood builder; it aids new growth; it regulates red blood cell formation and formation of genetic materials.

Deficiencies can result in pernicious anemia, parasthesia (temporary numbness), memory, and mental health problems. Vegetarians who eat no meat, milk, or eggs can become deficient in B-12 and develop pernicious anemia.

VITAMIN B-COMPLEX B-complex includes all the B vitamins needed to produce energy and for normal functioning of the nervous and digestive systems.

Women taking birth control pills can be deficient in B-vitamins.

FOLIC ACID (FOLACIN) Its name comes from the word *foliage*, because folic acid is found in green leafy vegetables, such as spinach. It is also found in organ meats such as kidney, liver, beef heart; lamb, pork, and chicken; brewer's yeast; asparagus; bran; tuna.

It interacts with B vitamins and vitamin C.

Folic acid is needed for production of healthy red blood cells. It is also synthetically made in the body in small amounts.

Deficiency can result in pernicious anemia and disorders in cell and tissue reproduction. Women who become pregnant after having been on birth control pills often have a folic acid deficiency.

VITAMIN C (ASCORBIC ACID, CALCIUM ASCORBATE)

Vitamin C is found in fresh vegetables and fruits, especially citrus, such as cantaloupe, cherries, strawberries, guava, tomatoes, parsley, green peppers, cabbage, broccoli, brussels sprouts, and potatoes.

It interacts with all vitamins and minerals, such as calcium and magnesium.

Vitamin C helps in healing; production of red blood cells and infection-fighting white blood cells; formation of bones, teeth, and cartilage; production of various hormones; and regulation of cholesterol. It also helps the body absorb iron and is said by some to help prevent stomach cancer.

Deficiency in vitamin C may result in hemorrhaging and edema (swelling), easy bruising, fatigue, infections, and sometimes complications following colds. Vitamin C deficiency can also cause poor dental health.

VITAMIN D This is found in fish liver oil, seafood such as tuna, salmon, herring; egg yolk; milk, cheese, and yogurt.

It interacts with vitamins A and C, calcium, and phosphorus. Called the "sunshine vitamin," it interacts with body oils when the sun hits the skin.

Vitamin D is needed to build strong bones and teeth, protect you from viral infections and muscular weakness. It's important in utilization of calcium and phosphorus in the body and helps regulate the heart because of calcium absorption.

Deficiencies in this vitamin can result in softening bones and teeth in adults, retarded and defective skeletal growth in children.

VITAMIN E (TOCOPHEROL) Vitamin E is found in most vegetable oils, all seeds and nuts, wheat germ, egg, beef liver, other meats, milk, molasses, legumes and green leafy vegetables, unrefined cereal products.

It interacts with vitamins A, B, and C, manganese, and selenium. Its name, tocopherol, means "oil of fertility" and comes from *tokos*, Greek for childbirth; *pherein*, which means "bring forth"; and *ol* for oil.

Vitamin E is said to improve muscle function by aiding oxygen flow to muscles, improve circulation, extend the life of red blood cells, prevent formation of blood clots, and reduce fatigue. Vitamin E also is said to increase sexual appetite, but I've been told there is not enough data available to prove this. In fact, some researchers say an overdose of vitamin E can actually decrease sex drive.

Deficiencies in vitamin E can cause hemolytic anemia in premature infants. Many other claims are made about the effects of vitamin E deficiency, but again, not all can be proven.

Research shows that it is nearly impossible to become deficient in vitamin E, even in laboratory experiments, but it is possible to overdose, and the result of vitamin E overdose can include headaches, low blood sugar, and upset stomachs.

VITAMIN K This is found in green leafy vegetables, kelp, milk, yogurt, egg yolks, and polyunsaturated oils.

Vitamin K is necessary for blood clotting, liver function, and healthy long life.

Deficiencies could result in easy bruising and blood-clotting abnormalities. Deficiency can also occur in people who have liver diseases.

Minerals

The best way to get enough minerals is to drink plenty of water and eat fresh, lightly cooked or raw foods. High heat removes some minerals. You should also avoid highly processed foods and sugary drinks.

Even the experts have not established the exact amounts of all minerals that we need daily. The National Academy of Sciences has a recommended dietary allowance (RDA) for six minerals and a standard of safe amounts to take for nine other minerals, but it's not known how much we need of minerals such as cobalt, nickel, and sulfur.

What is known is that the body controls minerals efficiently by itself and the only two minerals that occasionally become deficient are iron and calcium. Unless pregnant or nursing, only 10 percent of all women truly need iron supplements. Some young children and adolescents occasionally need iron, but most people get enough iron in their diets. Calcium deficiency is not the only cause of osteoporosis (weak, brittle bones) in elderly women; estrogen deficiency and physical inactivity also contribute to the disease.

CALCIUM   This is found in milk and milk products, dry kidney beans, potatoes, green vegetables, beef liver, whole grains, and unrefined cereals.

Calcium helps to build strong bones and teeth, calm nerves, promote normal blood clotting, and some research says it is necessary to maintain healthy heart action. In elderly women calcium deficiency, along with estrogen deficiency and lack of physical activity, contribute to the development of osteoporosis (brittle bones).

CHROMIUM   Brewer's yeast and spices are the best sources of chromium. It's also found in meats, liver, clams, unsaturated fats, and whole-grain cereals.

Chromium helps your body use carbohydrates and metabolize glucose properly. It also aids in the synthesis of fatty acids and cholesterol.

COPPER   Copper is found in most seafoods, liver, green leafy vegetables, whole-grain products, almonds and other nuts, and chocolate.

It is needed for production of hemoglobin and red blood cells and proper bone development. Deficiency is rare. But too much can lead to vomiting and diarrhea.

IRON   This is found in lean meats and liver, eggs, whole-grain products, vegetables, fruits, nuts, seeds, and brewer's yeast.

You need iron for healthy blood and to resist disease. Iron deficiency (anemia) is often found in people who have other vitamin and mineral deficiencies.

MAGNESIUM   Magnesium is found in whole-grain products, brown rice, oatmeal, nuts, dry beans and peas, soy products, dark green vegetables.

It aids in nerve and muscle function and helps maintain healthy bones.

MANGANESE   This is found in egg yolks, whole-grain cereals and flour, dried fruit, sunflower seeds and other nuts, dried peas and beans, brewer's yeast, coffee and tea.

You need manganese to activate many enzymes in the body. Deficiency is rare.

PHOSPHOROUS   It's found in all foods.

Phosphorous helps the body use proteins, carbohydrates, and fats properly; it also helps repair cells and produce energy. It's important for healthy bones and teeth, kidney function, and a healthy nervous system.

POTASSIUM   Meat and milk are good sources of potassium. It's found also in bananas, oranges, vegetables (especially those that are green and leafy), potatoes (especially in the peels), whole grains, and sunflower seeds.

You need potassium for healthy muscles, nerves, heart, and mineral balance in the blood. Potassium works with sodium to regulate your body's water balance. Sometimes people who take diuretics (water pills) develop potassium deficiencies that cause them to need supplemental potassium, but this is a decision for a physician to make. Some water pills have potassium among their ingredients to prevent such deficiencies.

SELENIUM   This is found in meats and seafood, milk and egg yolks, bran and cereals (although much of the selenium is lost in the milling process), broccoli, onions, tomatoes.

Selenium protects membranes from oxidative damage (wearing out) and aids the body's metabolism. Selenium is important to animals' enzyme systems and is considered important to humans, too.

ZINC Zinc is found in beans, nuts and seeds, oatmeal, wheat germ, seafood, liver, and other meats.

It is needed for new cell growth and healing, and it also aids digestive enzymes and metabolism. Zinc aids the reproductive system and normal functioning of the prostate gland. Getting too little zinc can affect your ability to taste. Taking too much zinc over a period of time can cause nausea and vomiting. Although whole grains contain zinc, they also contain a substance called phytate, which binds zinc and makes it less absorbable by the body.

Best Buys

Here are some of the most vitamin- and mineral-packed foods you can buy for your supermarket dollar:

- *Beans:* dry kidney beans are a super source of seven nutrients, especially vitamin B-6, protein, and calcium.
- *Beef liver:* liver provides eleven nutrients, and it's especially rich in vitamins A and B-12, riboflavin, and calcium.
- *Eggs:* despite cholesterol in the egg yolk, moderate eating of eggs (two or three a week) will provide nine nutrients, especially protein, vitamin B-12, and riboflavin.
- *Milk:* low-fat milk is a great nutritional buy because it provides ten nutrients, especially calcium, riboflavin, protein, and vitamin B-12.
- *Oatmeal:* it's still the most nutritious cereal available, providing at least a dozen nutrients, especially magnesium, thiamine, and zinc.
- *Peanut Butter:* a serving of peanut butter provides at least eight nutrients, including protein.
- *Potatoes:* potatoes contain at least twenty nutrients, especially vitamins C and B-6, calcium, and niacin.
- *Rice:* brown rice provides at least ten nutrients, especially magnesium, vitamin B-6, niacin, and thiamine.
- *Wheat Germ:* wheat germ is loaded with nine nutrients that can provide 100 percent of your daily requirements.
- *Whole-Wheat Bread:* It provides ten nutrients, especially thiamine, protein, and niacin.

• *Yogurt:* people who are unable to digest milk need not be denied its nutrients. Research has shown that yogurt can be a good substitute because it produces a milk-sugar-metabolizing enzyme for normal digestion that is lacking in those people who are unable to break down lactose (milk sugar) and suffer from bloating or diarrhea when they drink milk or eat other milk products.

• DIET-WISE TIPS •

Begin a Diet When You Are Most Likely to Succeed

The best time for a woman to start a diet is just after her menstrual period. If you start just before or during your period, you'll have to fight premenstrual food cravings, zero morale because you feel fat due to water retention and/or constipation, and a reluctance to exercise to help burn up your calories. But remember, you shouldn't stop dieting just because your period is due. Keeping your calorie count and salt intake down, adding fiber to your diet, and exercising more may actually reduce some of your menstrual distress. Getting slimmer is surely a good cure for any depression, and you can consider the usual three-to-five-pound water-weight gain a "plateau" in your diet.

Some experts suggest that you yield to your premenstrual food cravings for a day or two; but be sure to count calories so you won't really blow your whole diet while you improve your disposition.

Don't Eat When You Are Really Thirsty

How often do you wander around the kitchen, poke around in the refrigerator, and sneak snacks, when your body's real message is "I'm thirsty"? And the best lo-cal, free, and satisfying response to that kitchen craving call is a nice, big glass of water. Many weight-loss specialists recommend as many as eight or more glasses of water daily, and studies show that dieters who drink lots of water lose weight and feel less hungry than dieters who don't increase their water intake. Unlike other diet aids, you can't hurt your body with too much water, because your kidneys get rid of it.

Water flushes out the waste products from your body, and for people on low-carbohydrate diets, it helps prevent ketosis. Ketosis is a condition that can accompany low-carbohydrate diets when the body burns fat rapidly because it doesn't get its main energy source, carbohydrates. In ketosis, incompletely burned fat by-products go into the bloodstream where they cause extreme fatigue, constipation, and bad breath.

Read Labels

Look out for hidden sugar. It sneaks into seemingly innocent foods. Since ingredients are listed according to the amount contained in the product, if sugar is one of the first ingredients on a label, you may be getting more sugar in that product than you think. Sugar sneaks into catsup, many canned and processed foods, and breakfast cereals. When fruits such as peaches are canned in heavy syrup, there can be as much as 3.5 teaspoons of sugar in just one peach with a tablespoon of syrup.

Remember, sugar by any other name is still sugar, so watch out for: sucrose, zylose, fructose, mannose, corn sweetener, disaccharides, or monosaccharides.

Don't Skip Breakfast

Some people really can go without breakfast, but many more, especially those with low blood sugar, get tired, headachy, and are less able to function efficiently when their blood sugar drops from the overnight fast and no breakfast. If you skip breakfast, it's hard to resist stuffing down a sweet roll or other high-calorie snacks when you take your morning coffee break.

I eat bran and wheat germ for breakfast. To save both calories and fat, I don't pour milk on my cereal; I make my morning coffee with low-fat creamer; cool it; then pour it over the wheat germ. I think the coffee flavor is great and, best of all, I'm hardly adding any calories or fat.

Cut Back on Your Salt Intake

Studies show that eating too much salt throughout your life appears to change your body's reaction to restriction of salt. If you have always used lots of salt and are trying to get changes in blood pressure through salt restriction, you'll have to restrict your salt intake more severely than people who haven't used a great deal of salt throughout their lives.

You can learn to use other spices such as rosemary, basil, thyme, oregano, or lemon/lime juice to season your food. Soy sauce is also salty, but you can substitute beer or wine in recipes calling for soy sauce.

Remember, you are trying to avoid sodium, and ingredients other than table salt contain sodium, among them: MSG (monosodium glutamate), phosphates, nitrates, nitrites, and baking soda. Some products list the milligrams of sodium per serving; one that has more than 350 to 500 milligrams per serving should be considered a high-sodium food.

Foods high in sodium include: cured meats (ham, bacon, corned beef, luncheon meats, sausage); commercially frozen, breaded, fried, or smoked fish; any fish canned in oil or brine; canned shellfish; meat substitutes such as soy proteins; salted nuts; canned beans or peas; commercially prepared main dishes; instant cocoa mixes; cheeses; buttermilk; snacks such as chips or cookies; a variety of condiments, such as catsup, chili sauce, canned gravy, bouillon cubes, soy sauce, cooking wines, olives, pickles, bottled salad dressings, mayonnaise, and meat tenderizers. (Seems like just about everything!)

Reduce Your Fat Intake

Excessive use of any fat has been linked to breast and colon cancer in women; animal fats, which are high in saturated fats, also contain cholesterol, which clogs arteries. Saturated fats are contained in coconut oil or palm oil and hydrogenated vegetable shortening. Shortening usually means animal or vegetable fat, and liquid vegetable oil means polyunsaturated fat. One rule of thumb is: saturated fat is solid, and polyunsaturated fat is not.

Margarine is unsaturated fat. It has the same number of calories as butter, but low-fat margarine is lower in total fats.

SUITABLE SUBSTITUTES Margarine can be substituted for butter or lard; skim for whole milk; evaporated milk for cream; skim milk or low-fat cheese for whole-milk cheese; low-fat yogurt or cottage cheese, which has been whirred to smoothness in a blender or food processor, for sour cream; egg substitutes or one egg white and two teaspoons polyunsaturated oil for a whole egg; three tablespoons cocoa powder and one tablespoon polyunsaturated oil for one ounce of baking chocolate.

MORE SAVING WAYS   Let soups and stews cool, then remove fat from the top, and reheat them.

Steam or broil the foods you usually fry. Use vegetable spray or "fry" in bouillon instead of in fat.

Buy good or choice meat grades instead of prime, which has more marbling fat. And when you serve meat, slice it thin.

I think Butter Buds are a godsend. I mix up a package as per directions and add it to an almost finished tub of diet margarine, then add a drop of butter-flavor extract. I use this instead of butter and enjoy the taste of butter, with only one-tenth of the calories and fat. It's my favorite baked potato topping—I feel like I'm sinning when really I'm only downing about 120 calories!

Don't Get Fat "for Shame"

When you buy sweet treats for your family, buy only enough for one serving each so that you won't be tempted to eat the last piece of cake just because it would be "a shame" to let it dry out. Cook main courses in amounts that don't leave you leftovers to "clean up" because it's a shame to throw them out or a shame to reheat such a little bit for another meal.

Dietitian Judy New always tells folks who worry about "starving Armenians" to mail the food there. You don't have to eat for the world!

When you have a party, give the leftover food to folks who don't like to cook, or just give them to anybody who will take them—anyone, so long as you won't be tempted to eat them because it's a shame to waste such good food.

Collect Ideas for Low-cal Treats

Diet gelatin is one of my mainstays; so is the new hot chocolate made with Nutrasweet, even if the chocolate sometimes seems too sweet. Here's how I cut the sweetness: I mix the chocolate with almost twice the water recommended on the package; add a dash of rum or vanilla flavoring; and get two cups for the price of one—calorie-wise, that is.

Here are a few hundred-calorie or less snacks that you can use to soothe your hunger pangs (but remember to add the calories to your total for the day, and limit the liquor snacks to twice weekly).

SIP Try one cup skim milk; a six-ounce can of tomato, apple, or orange juice (unsweetened juices, remember); six ounces low-cal cocoa; six ounces light Chablis; four ounces dry champagne; six ounces light beer; eight ounces tonic water; coffee (better de-caf if you can do it); tea; consommé. Put lots of ice in your drinks to make them last longer for sipping. And drink water in between "flavored" drinks.

Beware: alcohol, like other sweets, may be habit forming, especially if you are the type who has trouble stopping after two Oreo cookies. Club soda is cheaper and lower cal than any alcoholic drink; order it with a twist or a dash of bitters for cocktails. It's even cheaper than prestige mineral bubbly waters and, some say, tastes about the same.

MUNCH Try four ounces shrimp cocktail; six raw clams or ten raw oysters; two cups raw veggies; two Oreo cookies; one low-fat frozen yogurt bar; one tablespoon chunky peanut butter (on celery or lettuce leaf, if you wish); one large mango or papaya; two cups unadorned popcorn; ten melba toast rounds; four large prunes; half a cup low-fat plain yogurt; eight potato chips; an orange; a hard-boiled egg; a medium banana; an apple; half a bran muffin or bagel (without butter).

Put a Freeze on Your Diet

Freeze leftovers so that you won't be tempted to finish them off, and freeze them in one-portion servings so that you can thaw yourself a proper-size meal. You can freeze diet foods for yourself and thaw a single portion for when your family is eating that rich quiche.

Eating Out and Traveling

Don't be afraid to call ahead and ask your airline about arranging to get a special meal. Some airlines will give you a fresh fruit or seafood plate if you ask for low-cal; some will give you a salad or vegetables if you order vegetarian; and an order for low-salt, low-cal might get you a broiled chicken plate.

Appetizers

In restaurants, order an appetizer that takes a long time to eat—soup or an artichoke—so you'll have something to do while the others gorge. Often the appetizers on the menu are better tailored to your diet than the entrées. There is no rule against ordering two appetizers or an appetizer and salad and no entrée.

And don't forget about that old favorite—the doggie bag! Take along a zip bag for your leftovers and enjoy them the next day. After all, you're paying for the dinner!

And while you're at it, pick a restaurant for lunch that is a comfortable walking distance away so that you'll burn up some calories walking to and from it instead of driving your car or taking a taxi to its door. Remember, twenty city blocks equal a mile! Or take your lunch to work and don't buy any snacks; you'll save money and calories!

Party Eating

Talk instead of eating. Sip instead of gulping. Pick instead of gorging. Eat your diet foods before you leave home if you are weak willed. Move yourself or the bowl of peanuts to avoid temptation. Try not to look at the dessert, and explain that dinner was so good that you'll just have coffee for dessert. Find someone at the party who is also trying to lose weight and make a pact to police each other.

Make Dieting Easier for Yourself

Instead of dessert, treat yourself to your "just desserts" as a reward for sticking to the diet—get a new hairstyle, a manicure, a facial. Avoid negative people who drag you down and depress you, which will send you running to the fridge. Find interesting things to do so that you feed your mind instead of your tummy. An expanded mind is much more attractive than an expanded tummy, right?

Make Rules

Tape a card to the fridge and write down when and what you cheated on so you'll remember not to do it again. Don't eat out of habit, such as before bedtime or when reading or test-tasting as you cook, and make some rooms and places off limits to food, especially the room with the TV. Also, don't eat standing up; eat only when you are seated at the table or kitchen counter, with a plate and silverware.

Chewing

Try chewing each mouthful twenty or thirty times, and stop to put your fork down occasionally. Do anything that makes you eat more slowly so that your body can have the twenty minutes it takes for your brain to get the message from your tummy that food is being processed. If you allow twenty minutes to pass, hunger will go away and you won't feel like gorging.

Plates

Use a smaller plate and spread food around so it looks like more. And drop out of the clean-the-plate club to join the unclean-plate club. Leave a little behind. You can do it—and you'll feel proud of yourself if you do.

Serve food from the stove on individual plates instead of family style, which tempts you to have seconds. Close up your kitchen after dinner; turn off the lights.

Make your diet meal special: use your good china, crystal, and silver if you are dining alone so that you feel as if you are having a treat instead of a treatment. I always set the table even if it's only me and a salad.

When Not to Eat

- Just because the food is there and looks nice.
- Because you don't know when you'll be eating later in the day and you want to avoid even the possibility of feeling hungry.
- When you are using food to make yourself feel good—less angry, lonely, afraid, unhappy, or any other emotion.
- Don't eat just because you are happy!

Slim Eating

Rate food and don't eat it unless it rates highly for taste, color, texture, and preparation. Be a gourmet and even a bit snobbish so you don't waste calories on food that doesn't give you pleasure.

Many people get fat because they will shovel in any edible morsel. Before you eat, stop; think about the food; rate it; then reject it if it doesn't get a good rating. (Try not to rate food aloud at a fancy dinner party—it's not likely to make you a popular guest. Rate silently; make it your secret system.)

Seasonings

Jazz up your diet foods with lemon or lime juice, herbs and spices you've never tried before, low-salt soy sauces, horseradish. Try some of the new flavored vinegars on your salad, and you may discover you don't need the oil in vinegar-and-oil dressing. Flavor with wine; a five-ounce glass of wine has approximately 125 calories, but when cooked the alcohol evaporates, adding only about 11 calories—and a lot of good taste.

Brush Your Teeth

Try brushing your teeth before you cook so you won't be tempted to taste; also brush your teeth before you settle down in front of the TV so you won't get up and use food as your entertainment. When you want a snack brush your teeth again, just for the taste of it.

Shopping

Don't shop when you're hungry. Avoid the center aisles of the supermarket, where all the caloric untouchables are displayed. Stick to your shopping list. Put all groceries in the trunk so you won't be tempted to sneak a munch on the way home.

Store Foods

Keep tempting foods out of sight in opaque containers. Freeze the ones that tempt you most.

Get Help

Have someone else clean up the kitchen so you won't be tempted to feed on the leftovers.

Look for Hidden Calories

Scrape off the breading on fried restaurant foods (or better yet, don't order them). I've been known to "peel" a whole batch of fried mushrooms. And just because a whole head of lettuce only has 56 calories, you don't have to add 500 calories worth of oil, bacon, sunflower seeds, croutons, grated cheese, and the like.

Don't Give Up

You need to decide what you'll eat for the day and stick to your decision, but if you slip up a bit, don't give up and think that you might as well pig out and start again tomorrow, the next day, or the next week. Forgive yourself the mistake and continue to diet.

When to Weigh

Many people weigh themselves once a week, but I prefer to weigh myself daily (before breakfast and after eliminating) so that I can watch my weight closely. Remember, a dieting lapse may not show up for two days.

Cutting Down

Did you know that if you eat 1 extra piece of chocolate cake (365 calories) every week you can gain 5 pounds a year?

But if you cut out 1 cake doughnut (2 ounces, about 230 calories) a day or 30 a month you can lose 24 pounds a year?

By cutting out 1 pat of butter or margarine on your potato (35 calories, 60 pats a month) you can lose 7 pounds a year.

Cut out 15 potato chips (1-ounce bag, 170 calories, 30 bags a month) and you'll lose 17 pounds in a year.

Give up sugar and nondairy coffee or tea creamer (1 teaspoon each, 25 calories, 90 cups a month) and you'll lose 8 pounds a year.

Cut out 1 can of beer (12 ounces, 150 calories, 30 cans a month) or 1 can of cola (12 ounces, 145 calories, 30 cans a month) and you'll lose 15 pounds *each* in a year.

Finally (sorry to be so un-American!), give up 1 slice of apple pie (5.6 ounces or one-eighth of a 9-inch pie, 300 calories, 8 pieces a month) and you'll lose 8 pounds a year.

I've probably lost any friends I might ever have had in the vending-machine business, because I'm afraid that's where you'll find most of the above items. If you dropped them all, you would lose 94 pounds in a year—probably more than you need to lose, but it proves how little you really have to give up to reach your goal.

• *DIET FACTS AND FANCY* •

We all have our own special "cures" and favorite health diets, often passed down from our grandmothers. Some are beneficial, others have been proven by recent research to be of little value, and some have even been proven harmful.

Not too long ago, I read about a woman who thought she was on a natural diet that would make her healthy and slim because she drank at least one pot of a "natural" herb tea daily. When she went to her doctor for treatment of abnormal menstrual bleeding, she discovered that it was her "health" herb tea (which contained tonka beans, melilot, and woodruff—all natural coumarin drugs) that was causing the abnormal bleeding.

The moral of this story? Don't play doctor by loading your body with megadoses of *anything* that is a fad "health food." Get as much information as possible about diets and other food supplements, natural or otherwise.

Antacids

Myth: antacids are harmless; that's why they're sold over the counter without a prescription. Take them to ease hunger pangs when you are dieting.

Fact: antacids help indigestion, but, when abused, compounds such as aluminum hydroxide can deplete the body of its nutrients.

Athlete's Food

Remember when Sylvester Stallone, in the movie *Rocky*, ate raw eggs while preparing for his fight? Other athletes eat red meat or drink protein powders or special tea concoctions. But many dietitians believe that the main benefit from ritualistically eating specific foods for strength is psychological. The mind says it's magic and the body believes and responds with a burst of energy that makes the athlete train harder, get into better physical condition, and maintain a winning attitude.

When an athlete takes in excessive amounts of protein, vitamins, and minerals, he or she risks overloading the liver and kidneys. When fat-soluble vitamins, such as A, D, E, and K, accumulate in the body, they can reach toxic levels that endanger health. Taking excessive B vitamins or C is a waste of money because unneeded amounts of these vitamins are excreted in the urine.

Bone Meal

Myth: bone meal is a great way to add calcium to your diet.

Fact: bonemeal (crushed animal bones) and dolomite (a stone) are found in health food stores and promoted as calcium sources, but they also are potentially dangerous sources of lead, which can lead to lead poisoning and/or leukemia. Most bone meal comes from horse bones, which accumulate and hold lead. The older the horse, the more lead. Older horses are sent to glue factories, which is where most bone meal is processed. It's claimed that the source of some bone meal is beef cattle, but there is no proof that beef bones have less lead than horse bones.

Bran

Myth: bran is a wonder food; the more you eat the better.

Fact: eating too much bran, like eating too much of any nutrient, can have a harmful effect on your body chemistry. Large amounts of bran can bind with iron in the body and carry it right through the digestive tract before the body can absorb the iron it needs. My dietitian says twenty-five to fifty grams of dietary fiber is okay. (One-half cup of a leading bran cereal equals about ten grams of dietary fiber.)

Bread and Potatoes

Myth: bread and potatoes are diet enemies and must be eliminated from your diet if it is to be successful.

Fact: bread and potatoes play a role in a reducing diet because of the nutrients they provide; it's what you add to them that ups the calorie count. One slice of bread is about 70 calories, but with one pat of butter or margarine, the calorie count goes up to 105. One medium baked potato is 105 calories, but with one pat of butter or margarine and two tablespoons of sour cream, the calorie count goes up to 190.

Caffeine

Caffeine is one diet addition that has been proven to physically benefit athletes. Some tests have shown that athletes who drink two and a half cups of coffee one hour before exercising have greater endurance—could continue moderate exercise for one-sixth more time than they could without caffeine. The reason? It's thought that caffeine increases the blood's fat levels, so the fat is used for energy and the glycogen (carbohydrates stored in the body) is saved for prolonged exercise.

The catch-22 in using caffeine for endurance: people who have a high tolerance for caffeine because they normally take in large amounts won't notice any difference in their endurance levels. And those who don't normally take in large amounts of caffeine sometimes get nausea and tremors—common reactions to large amounts of caffeine.

Calories

Myth: calorie counts are the same for equal amounts of all foods whether they are fats, proteins, or carbohydrates.

Fact: one ounce of fat contains 255 calories; one ounce of protein contains 113 calories; one ounce of carbohydrates contain 113 calories. One ounce of butter has more than twice the calories of one ounce of the baked potato you are drenching it with. So avoid food high in fat!

Cancer

Myth: there are no changes that you can make in your diet to prevent cancer.

Fact: studies at the National Cancer Institute indicate that a diet change in midlife may protect you from cancer. The studies comparing American diets, which are as much as 45 percent fat, to Oriental diets, which are about 15 percent fat, revealed that the rate of breast and colon cancer in China and Japan is only one-fifth of the cancer rate in the United States. Studies show, too, that eating more fresh fruits and vegetables—especially citrus fruits and vegetables of the cabbage family, is linked to a decline in cancer rates.

According to the American Cancer Society, smoking contributes to 30 percent of cancers, diet to 35 percent. The society suggests:

• Maintaining proper weight and cutting down on your total fat intake

• Eating more high-fiber fruits, vegetables, especially cruciferous vegetables like cabbage, broccoli, brussels sprouts, kohlrabi, cauliflower, and whole-grain cereals
• Eating foods rich in Vitamins A and C
• Drinking alcoholic beverages in moderation.

Sodium nitrite, which is used for color and preservation of fish and cured meats, such as ham or sausage, combines with other chemicals in the body to produce nitrosamines, some of which have been known to cause cancer. Some studies show that adequate vitamin C may decrease cancer risks due to nitrosamines, yet other research suggests that vitamin C blocks nitrosamine production in the stomach.

DES (diethylstilbestrol) has been linked to a rare form of cervical and vaginal cancer in young women whose mothers, while pregnant and threatened with miscarriage, were treated with DES. DES is used to fatten beef cattle and since diets high in fat have been shown to be linked with DES-caused cancer in animals and coronary artery disease in humans, cutting back on fat, instead of eliminating beef entirely from the diet (which may be difficult for some people), may decrease the risk of DES diseases. Try to eat only lean cuts of meat and remember that hamburger should contain less than 15 percent fat.

Carbohydrates

Myth: to save calories while dieting, cut out as many carbohydrates as you can.

Fact: Although it's true that too many carbohydrates—sugars and starches—will give you lots of calories and added pounds, beware of a very low-carbohydrate diet. It may cause your scale to register a quick weight loss because cutting carbohydrates causes water loss, but water loss is not fat loss. Carbohydrates are involved in helping the body use protein. Too few carbohydrates can harm the kidneys, lower blood pressure, and cause headaches, weakness, and dizziness (ketosis).

Cottage Cheese

Myth: cottage cheese is a diet food.

Fact: regular cottage cheese contains a moderate amount of fat and is not low in calories, but it often shows up on restaurant diet plates. Choose skim-milk cottage cheese for your reducing plan.

Diet and Age

Myth: as long as you don't eat more than you ate when you were in your twenties, you *can* maintain your twenties figure.

Fact: your metabolism slows down as you get older. If you needed 1,350 calories a day when you were in your twenties, you'll only need about 1,300 in your forties (depending on individual metabolic and activity levels), and those extra 50 calories a day will increase your weight by one to three pounds a year. Gaining one to three pounds a year doesn't sound like much, but multiplied by ten or twenty years, it's a pretty sobering thought! The solution is, of course, to change your eating habits as you get older to eliminate 80 calories a week between your twenties and thirties; eliminate 200 calories a week if you are over thirty, and you will stay the same weight as you were in your twenties. But if you are a few pounds overweight, you'll need to cut out an additional 25 to 30 calories a day to be two or three pounds lighter. (These figures are based on a five foot, four inch tall, 120-pound woman.)

Diet Pills

Myth: nonprescription diet pills, which are sold over the counter, are safe for everyone.

Fact: nonprescription diet pills contain phenylpropanolamine (PPA) and benzocaine, which cut your appetite but do nothing to change your eating habits. PPA is not safe for people with heart disease, hypertension, diabetes, or thyroid problems, and it's dangerous for pregnant women. Read the fine print on the label.

Prescription diet pills contain amphetamines, but after six or eight weeks, you can develop a tolerance to them so they won't work. You also may develop an addiction to them. Some people react to amphetamines with nervousness, hallucinations, nausea, upset stomach, sleeplessness, or paranoia.

You may lose weight by taking diet pills, but you may damage your health in the process—and for naught, as it's unlikely you'll keep the weight off, because a pill can't teach you new eating habits.

Exercise

Myth: exercise makes you hungrier and then it's harder to diet.

Fact: in addition to improving muscle tone, circulation, and heart strength, exercise actually helps control your appetite. Some people find that they can exercise instead of snacking and not crave nibbles at all.

Fat

Myth: saving calories by cutting all or as much as possible of the fat from your diet is a good idea.

Fact: know why you feel hungry an hour after eating in your favorite Oriental restaurant? Chinese food doesn't contain enough fat to slow down digestion and keep you feeling full longer.

Fat is necessary to carry fat-soluble vitamins A, D, E, and K from your digestive tract to your tissues, and fatty acids are absolute essentials in your diet. Fat also insulates your body and provides padding for your organs. We all know that too much fat equals too much padding, but 30 percent of our daily calories should be in the form of fat.

Food Additives

Myth: beware of food additives—they're all dangerous.

Fact: additives are not all chemical mysteries. Many are actually natural food compounds and some are produced in the body. For example, calcium propionate, used to prevent mold in our bread, is found naturally in Swiss cheese and is also produced in the body. Citric acid is naturally found in citrus fruits. Beet coloring is used in some foods. The most commonly used additives are sugar (sucrose), corn sweeteners (corn syrup, dextrose, and fructose), and salt (sodium chloride).

Fruit

Myth: fruit is a low-calorie snack.

Fact: canned fruits often have sugar added. Choose those that are packed in their own juice. Also, some fruits are higher in calories than others. Choose the lowest in calories, such as grapefruits and oranges. Actually, raw vegetables are best for the nibbles.

Gelatin

Myth: gelatin is pure protein and therefore a good energy source, as well as a nail strengthener.

Fact: gelatin powder is pure protein, but it lacks the essential amino acids, so any other protein food is more useful to your body and your fingernails. Gelatin is no better an energy source than sugar.

Iron

Myth: all women need iron supplements as long as they are menstruating. Normal menses cause anemia.

Fact: although women lose iron when menstruating, it's estimated that only 10 percent have sufficient bleeding to lead to iron deficiency. Eating a well-balanced diet, including iron sources such as liver, eggs, meat, dried fruit, grains, and beans, should give most women the iron they need. Some women are sensitive to iron supplements and suffer digestive disturbances, such as diarrhea or stomachaches when taking them or when taking vitamin tablets with extra iron.

Kelp

Myth: kelp is one of the many sea products that miraculously makes us healthy. Kelp is especially good for healing bones and other tissues because it contains iodine.

Fact: overdoses of kelp tablets, taken by those who believe more is better, have caused arsenic poisoning and metabolism problems. Kelp is sometimes so rich in iodine that it can, with prolonged use, lead to thyroid and, subsequently, metabolism disorders.

Kids and Adults

Myth: skinny kids grow up to be skinny adults.

Fact: active children burn up a lot of calories, but if they are encouraged to eat sweets or fatty, high-calorie foods, they will develop poor eating habits and will grow up to be overweight adults no matter how thin they were as children.

Lecithin

Myth: take lecithin to dissolve cholesterol and/or keep it in an emulsion state in your body. Lecithin helps your body get rid of fat.

Fact: lecithin is naturally produced in the body and there is no need to take any supplemental doses. It does not dissolve cholesterol, keep it in emulsion, or dissolve the placque from your arteries to prevent atherosclerosis. One of the main benefits of lecithin, it seems, is that it's a real money-maker for those who sell it.

Milk

Myth: the reason milk at bedtime is so soothing is purely psychological; we are remembering our baby bottles.

Fact: milk contains a sleep-inducing amino acid called tryptophan. In addition to making people sleepy, tryptophan has been reported to make some people feel less depressed and others lose weight. Tryptophan also acts in the bloodstream to boost the amount of pain-relieving chemical called serotonin in the brain. Studies show that a diet that is 10 percent protein, 70 to 80 percent complex carbohydrates, accompanied by nutritional supplements containing tryptophan, helped people fight chronic pain. However, self-prescribing tryptophan supplements is not a good idea; consult a physician.

Papaya

Myth: the enzymes in papaya will somehow gobble up calories inside your digestive tract and you'll lose weight.

Fact: papaya enzymes tenderize meat—before it's cooked and long before it's eaten. Any enzyme that goes into your body through your mouth is destroyed by your stomach acids before it can exert any action in your digestive tract. Papaya won't magically make you thin.

Protein

Myth: protein is an important part of our diet. The more we take in the better.

Fact: studies of the American diet show that even at poverty level, we eat 60 to 100 percent more protein than we need. The average person gets three to five times as much protein as is required for health. Only 15 to 20 percent of our diet needs to be protein food.

Quick Weight Loss

Myth: the quicker you lose weight the better.

Fact: studies show that 90 to 95 percent of all diets fail because the faster you lose, the faster you regain. But failure is not the biggest problem. Very low-calorie diets deplete muscle mass; regaining the weight replaces fat deposits first, and in greater amounts than before. Gaining the weight back quickly also causes higher blood cholesterol levels and greater deposits of cholesterol in your blood vessels—dangerous to your cardiovascular system, which means an increased risk of heart disease. It is better to lose one or two pounds weekly and then adjust your life-style to keep it off.

Sea Salt

Myth: sea salt is much healthier than ordinary sodium chloride table salt because it contains super nutrients.

Fact: sea salt is no healthier than ordinary (and less expensive) table salt.

Snacks

Myth: you have to give up all snacks if you want to lose weight.

Fact: it's the total amount of food you eat each day that counts. Some people feel better if they eat "three squares a day," whereas others like four or five light meals a day. You should develop your own eating style, stay on a schedule, and keep track of the total calories eaten. Snacks, if they are low-calorie and nutritious, may actually help you stick to a lower-calorie regime by keeping your appetite from getting out of control. High-fiber snacks stay in the stomach longer and are good for this.

Sugar

Myth: substituting fructose or other sugars for table sugar is healthier for you.

Fact: the body doesn't care where its glucose for energy comes from. Carbohydrates become glucose; sugar becomes glucose; so does fructose; and the body uses the glucose no matter what the source. Also, extracting fructose from fruit is a very expensive process, so the fructose sold in most stores is taken from cornstarch instead. (Maybe it should be relabeled "starchtose.") But, since fructose tastes sweeter per unit than regular sugar, you may save calories because you'll use less per serving.

Whole Milk

Myth: whole milk is more nutritious than skim or low-fat milk.

Fact: although very young children may benefit from some milk fat, whole milk is not better for you than skim. Skim milk has all the nutrients of whole milk, but not the saturated fat or the calories.

• *EXERCISE: FINDING THE RIGHT PROGRAM FOR YOU* •

Before you read this section, try this:

1. Close your eyes (take off your glasses if you wear them).
2. Each time you inhale, count the odd numbers from one to nine (one, three, five, seven, nine), visualizing each number. Each time you exhale, count the even numbers from two to ten (two, four, six, eight, ten), visualizing each number. Start with one while inhaling, two while exhaling, until you have counted to ten. Inhale through your nostrils slowly; exhale through your mouth, and try to hold the air in for a count of five. You should feel as if you are filling up your lungs, stomach, even your throat, with air.
3. Open your eyes.

Wasn't that easy? You have just done a yoga-style exercise that is used by many dieters as a distraction to help avoid unnecessary munching. Whenever you feel like eating and you're not really hungry, do this exercise. It works. And did you notice how easy it was? Not all exercise leaves you sweaty and exhausted, and not all exercise is the kind that strengthens muscles. Some exercises strengthen your willpower!

While we're at it, here's my favorite exercise to prevent my going to the kitchen and eating when I'm not really hungry (I like to call this "nonfunctional eating"). Get up and walk to your kitchen, just as if you were going to sneak a snack. But instead of going to the fridge, walk to the cupboard, reach for a glass, fill it with water, and drink it down slowly. I bet you'll discover this really works. What's more, you'll be downing some of your eight-glass daily quota of water for better health.

Getting started on an exercise program is the most difficult part of the entire weight-loss experience. It's so easy to postpone, but if you are going to diet for better health and weight loss, you need to exercise, too, so that your body will firm up as it slims down.

Exercise is a proven stress reliever and, of course, cardiovascular/aerobic exercise is an absolute must for increasing your metabolism and unclogging your circulatory system.

Would you believe that some people think the need to exercise lessens after age fifty? The truth is that a regular exercise program —even just walking, stretching, and dancing—helps slow aging, whatever your age. It will also make you feel happier, more energetic, and less klutzy as your body discovers fitness.

• *STARTING UP A PROGRAM* •

The time to start is *now*, and here's how to do it:

Physical Checkup

If you are over thirty, overweight, or have ever had high blood pressure or heart trouble, you should have a complete physical examination before starting any sort of exercise program. Tell your doctor what you are planning to do; certain health problems determine the type of exercise that's best for you. For example, some doctors suggest that those who have high blood pressure should not do isometric exercises because the muscle-on-muscle pressure can raise blood pressure.

Listen to Your Body

When your body talks to you, listen. If you push yourself to the point of pain, you'll soon give up the whole program. Begin slowly and work up to greater activity levels gradually. Don't forget to warm up and cool down to prevent injuries and excessive pain.

Learn to distinguish between the pain of working muscles and the pain of injury. For example, a sudden, sharp pain usually means injury and is a plea from your body to ease up and/or avoid a particular movement.

Warming Up to Exercise

Warm up for *any* kind of exercise with five to ten minutes of bending and stretching to literally "get your heart and lungs started," and to warm or limber up your muscles. After working out, cool down or "warm down," as some say, by taking five to ten minutes of slow-down exercise to let your body return to its prestress condition.

I jog for ten to twenty minutes on a small trampoline for my aerobic exercise. If I don't warm up by slowly bouncing on the tramp or stretching, I sometimes get leg cramps while jogging. And believe me, if I don't do some warm-down stretches I feel so rubber-legged I have a hard time walking around the house!

If you are warming up to run, do five to ten minutes at a slower pace than usual, and warm down by easing into the same slower pace for five to ten minutes at the end of your run. Remember, it is the duration rather than speed of your activity that is important. You need at least twenty to thirty minutes of aerobic exercise for optimum results. If you can't run for twenty to thirty minutes straight, walk part of that time; the key is to keep moving constantly.

One of my research assistants, who says she has fifty years of nonexercising behind her (and on the front of her, too), has started running on the tramp. She says it took her three or four weeks of tramp jogging three to five times weekly to work up to twenty- or twenty-five minute sessions without getting red-faced or huffing and puffing. In the beginning, she gasped and panted so much after only ten to fifteen minutes that it made her dog bark in panic. Now she hates to miss a day and sometimes jogs twice daily—during the morning and evening news on TV.

Getting Hooked on the Habit

Get hooked on a regular form of exercise. The best habit, of course, is a daily one, but if you can't, exercise at least three to four times weekly for a minimum of twenty minutes, or better, thirty minutes each session. Many find a schedule of two twenty- to thirty-minute workouts during the week, plus weekend sessions that are twice as long, a very workable workout schedule.

Important: don't let yourself get bored with your exercise, so that you'll have an excuse to quit. Vary your routine. I find that jogging on a tramp while watching TV makes the time pass quickly. But when I exercise with my eyes fastened on my digital clock, sixty seconds seems like sixty minutes!

The Right Exercise Program for You

Find a program that suits your body, temperament, and schedule. Some like to have the support of a group when exercising; others prefer to go it alone. You can get help in putting together a fitness program from your local YWCA or YMCA, through adult education programs at local colleges and universities, and, more and more, from employers. Many companies are providing fitness programs for employees because it has been proven that healthy people are more productive.

Rating Spas or Health Clubs

Beware of clubs offering miracle programs that will "melt off fat" in a few days.

One of the "miracle" programs dubbed real baloney by the Food and Drug Administration is "passive exercise," wherein you're hooked up to a machine that gives electric shocks to your muscles, a procedure that supposedly exercises them with no exertion on your part. The fact is, electrical stimulation to contract muscles is a valuable tool used by physical therapists to help injured patients regain use of their limbs, but it has no slimming benefits.

When you find a health club that seems appealing, check out one of its exercise classes. Is it so crowded you will have trouble seeing the instructor? Mirrors on the ceiling help everyone get a good view.

Is the club really health conscious? By that I mean, is smoking allowed?

If you are interested in specific sports, does the club's flooring suit you? For example, do you like tennis courts with asphalt or sports carpeting; racquetball courts with oak or maple floors; jogging paths with gravel or cushioned running surfaces?

Will you be embarrassed if you have to undress to use the sauna or soak in a whirlpool with others, even wearing a swimsuit? At some spas, people do not wear swimsuits in the public areas and feel comfortable nude. Will you?

Is there a clock in good view of the hot tub, whirlpool, and sauna so that you will be able to time your soaking and steaming? Is there adequate instruction on easing into use of these facilities? Until your body is accustomed to the heat, steam, and swirling of the spa treatments, you may feel faint or at least like a limp noodle if you stay in too long. It's important not to overdo it, even *after* you are accustomed to such facilities.

And finally, can you really afford to join a health club? Often these clubs have discounted prices during special membership drives. This is a good time to try them out to see if you want to spend the money on full membership. If you can afford a health club, but feel guilty about spending the money to join one, remember that you can't put a price tag on fitness. You want the best fitness program, one that suits you and one that you will like enough to continue. If you don't enjoy it, you'll drop out and go right back to square one.

• TESTING YOUR FITNESS PROGRAM •

A good program has four major elements:

1. Cardiovascular Conditioning

Cardiovascular exercise makes your heartbeat stronger, your breathing deeper, and improves circulation. Improved circulation gives you more energy and increased awareness, and the experts say that exercise decreases the risk of heart disease. Exercises that strengthen the heart include jogging, bicycling, brisk walking, and dance/exercise, such as aerobic dance or jazz.

2. Tissue Flexibility

You need to stretch muscles and move your joints for better posture and to prevent your muscles and other connective tissues from losing their elasticity from disuse. Improving flexibility can reduce lower back pain for some people, and, of course, good posture makes you look and feel better. Stretching exercises, dancing, and swimming are good activities for increasing flexibility.

3. Endurance

As you get into your exercise program. you will gain muscular endurance, and you will be able to recover more rapidly from vigorous exercise and exercise longer before you feel tired. Jogging, brisk walking, cross-country skiing, bicycling, canoeing, and racquet sports increase endurance.

4. Strength

Muscular strength is useful for everything you do. It also helps your posture and, therefore, your appearance. Weight lifting is the best way to increase your strength, but calisthenics and aerobic dancing will also make you stronger. Many people think *all* weight lifters get huge, bulgy muscles, but that's not the case unless you go to extremes. A light weight-lifting program with proper supervision will improve muscular strength and tone, which means better posture, easing of lower back pain, and firmer stomach muscles. When you exercise, strong muscles get stronger, but weak muscles can be damaged if you don't have a sensibly balanced exercise program that deals with total body fitness.

• BUILD FITNESS •

If You Choose to Run

Find a pleasant place—a park, a trail, an interesting neighborhood (minus unfriendly dogs). Don't avoid hills—they give your thighs a better workout.

Your foot should land under your knee, your shoulders should be relaxed and down. Use your arms for balance by letting them move back and forth naturally. If you have never run before, don't expect to get out there and do three miles right off. Some people recommend "wogging"—a combination of walking several paces and jogging several paces, the number depending on your comfort zone, then working up gradually to a full jog. Remember, you're not in a race; find a comfortable pace and maintain it, but you don't have to go full tilt from first step to last!

If You Choose to Walk

Walking briskly is best. If you maintain a quick pace you'll be tightening up your buttocks and the backs of your thighs. Find a good hiking area so walking will be fun, or walk your dog, who probably needs exercise as much as you do. When you walk, roll your foot from your heel forward and push off your steps from the ball of your foot. Keep your head and body upright without leaning forward. If you keep your elbows bent racer style, you'll walk faster. If you have not done any walking for a long time, walk a quarter of a mile daily to start and increase gradually until you work up to two miles or more a day.

If You Choose to Bike

Get maximum benefit from biking either outdoors or on a stationary bike by "sprinting" occasionally. Outdoors you can enjoy fresh air and scenery, indoors on a stationary bike you can avoid boredom by watching TV, reading, listening to music, or doing anything else that keeps you interested.

I read about a man who connected a stationary bike to a generator that ran his TV. Anytime anyone in the family wanted to watch TV, someone had to pedal the bike. They took turns during shows the whole family watched. Not a bad idea.

When you are using any kind of bike, make sure the seat height is right for you. How to tell? Sit down and pedal; if your leg is almost fully extended and comfortable when the pedal is all the way down, it should be right. You can convert an ordinary bike to a stationary bike by buying a stand that raises the rear wheel and prevents it from going forward. This is called a turbo trainer.

If You Choose to Swim

Try snorkeling to make it more fun and switch strokes so that you won't get bored. The biggest calorie burner is the crawl.

If You Choose Aerobic Dancing

Take a class so you can learn the basic steps. Buy a tape to use while dancing. Dance in front of a mirror so you can see if you are doing the routines properly. Don't overdo it.

If You Choose to Ski

If you live in a climate where you can cross-country ski, learn to glide longer on each ski to cover longer distances faster. Use a pole for balance and forward thrust. Get instructions on proper form.

If You Choose to Skate

Wear protective pads on knees, elbows, and wrists, and if you really get into speed skating, wear a helmet. The best workout position is to lean forward, crouch down, and keep your head up. Let arms swing to keep you balanced—and burn more calories.

• CALORIE BURNUP •

You can find lots of charts about the number of calories different activities burn up, but I like the following general estimate from the President's Council on Physical Fitness and Sports. (The number of calories burned depends on your body frame and weight, that's why there's a range instead of specific number burned.)

Strenuous Activity

You'll burn 350 or more calories per hour in strenuous activities such as swimming, tennis, running, dancing, skiing, or football. Cycling at eight miles per hour (six for a beginner) is good aerobic exercise, and tennis, table tennis, badminton, or volley ball are good if the games provide vigorous continuous play for thirty minutes. Remember, swimming does not mean sitting in your pool. Jogging at five miles per hour burns up to 600 calories per hour; it also builds endurance.

Vigorous Activity

You'll burn 250 to 350 calories per hour in vigorous activities such as bowling, golfing, or gardening, but you won't get a thorough cardiovascular workout because you don't usually have a sustained activity level for the necessary twenty to thirty minutes. Nor do these activities promote endurance. Brisk walking means walking at three miles per hour, and is adequate cardiovascular exercise for a beginner. A moderate walking pace means about two miles per hour.

Moderate Activity

You'll burn 170 to 240 calories per hour with moderate activities such as walking at an average pace or playing Ping-Pong.

Light Activity

You'll burn 110 to 160 calories per hour for light activities such as walking slowly, ironing, or doing dishes. Isn't that a great excuse to get someone else to do the dishes and ironing so that you can go out and get some real cardiovascular exercise by walking briskly or jogging? You need the exercise!

Sedentary Activity

You'll burn up 80 to 100 calories per hour with sedentary activities such as reading, writing, watching TV, sewing, or typing.

· COMPUTING CALORIE NEEDS ·

Add up your calorie needs according to your weekly activities and then balance your food intake according to the number of calories you will need for your activity level.

Here's one way to compute your calorie needs. Some people allow one hundred pounds for the first five feet of their height and three to five pounds for each additional inch. This means that if you are five foot, ten inches, you should weigh 130 to 150 pounds, depending on whether you have a small, medium, or large frame.

Since a pound of stored fat (doesn't that sound awful?) contains 3,500 calories, to lose just one little pound, you need to cut out

3,500 calories from your regular calorie intake. For example, if you normally eat 2,000 calories daily, cut to 1,500 calories daily for seven days to lose one pound weekly. Most diet experts agree that a safe low-calorie intake is 1,200 per day.

• *FIRMER-UPPERS FROM HEAD TO TOE* •

Whether you do yoga, calisthenics, aerobics, isometrics, dancercises, or gym workouts; whether you jog, swim, or walk—whatever you do, chances are you will get as bored as I have with various routines. That's why I've collected these exercises from friends and other sources. When you get bored with one routine, try another that's suggested for the part of your body that's bored.

Here's my favorite yoga exercise. I think it's a good way to start a day.

First, relax by letting your head drop comfortably forward, then slowly roll your head completely around to the right and then to the left about three times.

Now, lift your shoulders up to your ears (even if you can't get them to touch), and let your shoulders drop; do this about five times.

Next, stand with your feet apart, and swing your right arm around in a circle about thirty times; do the same with your left arm. These swings will get blood circulating above your waist and make you feel more awake.

Here are some stretchercises to limber you up and some exercises to firm you up—from your top to your bottom.

• *STRETCHERCIZES* •

Remember to stretch and warm up before doing vigorous exercises so that you prevent injuries! The following is from my dear friend Laurie Hostetter, who owns and runs Kerr House in Grand Rapids, Ohio. I do it faithfully every morning.

Standing Triangle

Inhale, slowly stretching arms to shoulder height. Reach out as if trying to touch side walls with hands.

Exhale, bending to right side, arm over ear. Hold.

Inhale, up. Repeat on left side.

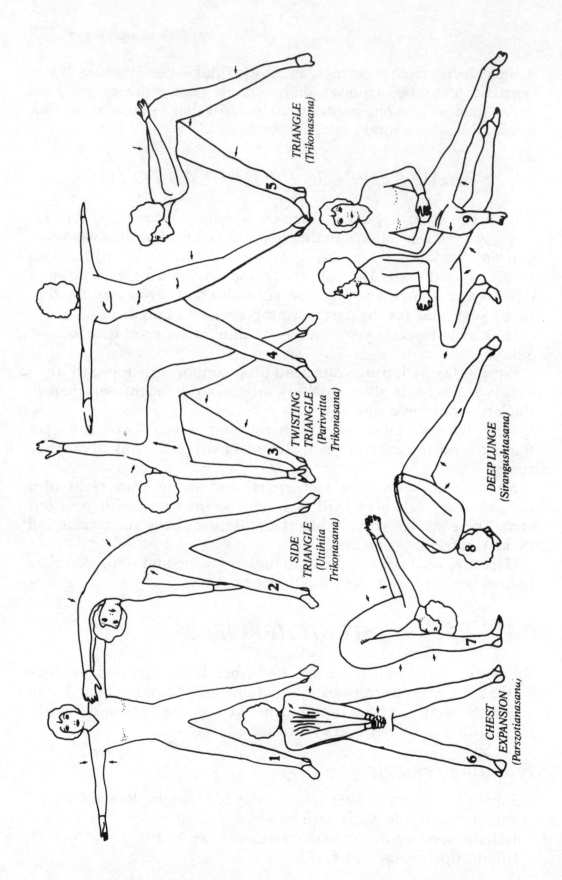

TRIANGLE
(Trikonasana)

TWISTING
TRIANGLE
(Parivritta
Trikonasana)

SIDE
TRIANGLE
(Uttihita
Trikonasana)

DEEP LUNGE
(Sirangushtasana)

CHEST
EXPANSION
(Parszotianasana)

Exhale, while slowly reaching for right leg or foot with left hand, twisting chest toward back wall. (Put pressure on your leg.) Hold. Inhale while returning to first position. Repeat on other side.

Exhale while twisting upper trunk from waist so you face back wall. Hold. Inhale while returning forward. Repeat on other side.

Relax. Take two deep inhalations and exhalations.

Exhale while bending from hips, reaching for your thigh with your rib cage, then tucking head to leg. Hold. Inhale, returning to first position. Repeat on other side.

Clasp hands behind back, pulling shoulder blades together and locking elbows. Arch slightly.

Exhale while slowly bending forward, stretching locked arms overhead. Inhale while returning to first position. Repeat on other side.

Relax. Take two deep inhalations and exhalations.

Spread legs far apart. Exhale while lowering head to toe in deep lunge. Inhale, up slowly. Repeat on the other side. Use your hands to avoid strain.

Point toes forward. Exhale as you slowly lean to your right, squatting on your right leg, keeping your left leg straight. Repeat on left side. Do not strain!

Benefits: stimulates circulation to heart, head, throughout body. Loosens tense muscles of back, shoulders, legs. Stretches spine, gives strength and flexibility to legs, ankles, and improves balance. Reduces abdominal fat and helps cure indigestion and constipation, tones up liver, kidneys, and pancreas. Excellent for muscle tone, weak back, good posture. The weak muscles of the sides are strengthened and tension removed by stretching. Seldom-used muscles of the thighs are toned. The slow movements combined with deep breathing and stretching work on cellulite areas.

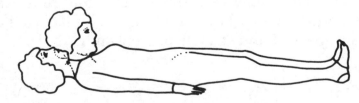

Head Lift

Position: Lie flat on back, legs together, heels pointed.

Inhale.

Exhale while lifting head slowly and placing chin on chest, pressing chin firmly into jugular notch Do not lift shoulders. Retain exhalation and lock. Hold.

Inhale while slowly returning head to floor. Hold air in. Push out. Repeat three times.

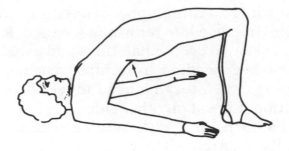

Hip Lift

Exhale while slowly bending knees and sliding feet to hips. Lock.

Inhale, raise hips off floor, keeping knees and feet together. The weight will be on the feet and shoulders. Relax shoulders, push body (with feet) toward shoulders to cause higher arch. Push out.

Exhale while slowly lowering body to floor, vertebra by vertebra. Lock

Repeat three times.

Benefits: head lift causes extension of spinal cord and nerve centers, releases tension in neck and shoulders, strengthens neck. The push-out increases circulation to the ear drums and sinuses and throughout the inner organs. Hip lift: muscles of legs, hips, spine, and ligaments are stretched. The locking of the anal sphincter is excellent for muscle tone.

Body

While lying on the floor (or a firm bed), stretch your entire body from the tips of your fingers to the tips of your toes to feel as tall as you can. Hold for five seconds; relax and repeat a few times, then stretch slowly in all directions until you feel as if every single muscle has moved and stretched. Easy, huh?

Body, Legs, Arms

Stand with your feet apart and your arms at your sides. Reach to touch the side or back of your right leg with your right hand, and bend and slowly slide as far down as you can; you can extend your left arm for balance; slide back up again. Repeat about six times and then do the same with the other hand and foot. I do this as slowly as possible.

Upper Body

Stand with your feet apart, arms at shoulder level. Alternate reaching for the ceiling with each hand, stretching toward the right with your left hand, and to the left with your right hand. Then reach out and try to touch the ceiling with both arms, swaying from side to side so that your waist notices what you're doing.

To do another upper-body exercise, lie down, with legs straight and arms raised; stretch fingers apart while you stretch both arms up to touch the ceiling. Slowly lower your arms to your sides, then stretch them back and forth making "angel wing" motions along the floor. Relax. Repeat if you wish.

Lower Body

Lying on the floor, raise your right knee to your chest and grasp it with both hands so that you can pull your knee as close to your chin as possible, keeping shoulders flat. Lower your right knee slowly, placing pressure against your hands. Repeat exercise with your left leg and relax.

Calves

To stretch calf muscles before running, stand about two feet from a wall, arms stretched forward at shoulder level, your palms resting on the wall. Then bend your arms as you lean toward the wall and step forward with your left foot. Keep your back straight. Press your right heel to the floor slowly and hold for fifteen seconds, then relax for three seconds. Do this stretch up to six times, then switch feet and repeat. This is the classic calf stretch done by many people before running or walking briskly.

Hamstrings

To stretch hamstrings, those tendons in the back of your knees, stand with your feet together and knees bent; then bend from the waist until you can touch your palms to the floor right there in front of your feet. If you haven't bent any part of your body recently except your elbow to hold a fork, just go as close to the floor as you can. After you bend, slowly straighten your legs, with your hands or fingertips still on the floor. Feel the stretch in your hamstrings. Go back to starting position, and repeat ten times. Once you are in good shape, you can vary this exercise by "walking your hands" until they are behind you and your chest touches your knees. But don't get discouraged—it takes a long time to get that limber!

To do another hamstring exercise, lie on the floor on your back, holding your arms at your sides, with your knees bent and your feet flat on the floor. As you push the small of your back to the floor and your hips upward, straighten one leg and lower to the floor, flexing your foot. Then slowly lift the straightened leg up until you can feel a pull in the back of your thigh. Hold this position for fifteen seconds, then lower your leg to the floor and return to your original position. Repeat with the other leg; work out each leg six times.

Office Stretchers

For a stretch you can do in your office chair, put your hands on your knees, and then slowly arch your back and tilt your head back as you stretch your spine and neck. Let your head fall slowly forward. Then, as you bend your elbows, curl your body forward, head going toward your lap. Return to an upright position slowly, with your tummy muscles tight and your shoulders relaxed. Then glance around your office to see if anybody's looking!

For another simple stretcher, simply stretch. Clasp your hands in front of you, fist-closed position; then change hands and stretch arms forward, up and back, for a mighty rib cage raising, back straightening, tummy tucking, backward stretch. Then pull slightly to the left; to the right; to the center. Stretch forward again, and back to original position. Hold each position for a few seconds. Repeat until you get enough air into your lungs to feel alert and refreshed.

For a third stretch, sit on your chair, feet flat on the floor; inhale slowly through your nose, imagining the breath filling up your stomach, then your chest and throat; then exhale slowly. Repeat several times and see how this yoga breathing takes the tension from every part of your body and lets you get through the day in better temperament. If you close your eyes it's more effective.

Legs

While lying on the floor, point your toes to the ceiling, stretching your foot from your ankle, and then rotate your foot at the ankle, describing about six circles in the air with your toes; then lower your leg slowly and repeat exercise with other leg. Relax; repeat if you wish.

To stretch inner thighs, sit on the floor Indian style, keeping your back straight and the soles of your feet pressed together. With your hands on your ankles and your elbows resting on your knees, lean forward and gently press your knees outward to the floor, holding the pressed position for about ten to fifteen seconds. Don't bounce. Try to keep your back flat. Release. Repeat five times or more.

To stretch front and outer thighs, sit on the floor, arms behind your buttocks, leaning slightly back and with your knees bent (the old glamor girl pin-up pose). Keeping your knees and feet together, but holding the rest of your body firm, press your knees to the right, keeping them together as they touch the floor; then press to the left, holding each "touch" for about fifteen seconds. Do each side about six times. I like to do these slowly.

Legs and Hips

While you are on the floor, with your legs straight and your arms at your sides, pull one knee up to your tummy, and then slowly slide your foot along the floor until your leg is straight again. Try not to slouch. Alternate legs on this stretch and do as many as make you feel comfortably relaxed and limber.

• TONERS AND TRIMMERS •

Arm Deflabber

Stand up straight, arms outstretched to sides at shoulder height. Flex hands and point fingers straight; make big circles with arms, first forward and then backward. This will also help your posture.

The following push-up will firm up arms and bosoms. With your arms extended, elbows straight, supporting your body weight, and your toes (or knees, with ankles crossed) touching the floor, lower your body slowly to the floor, keeping your knees, hips, chest, and shoulders in a straight line, with elbows bent and extended outward. Push back up. Inhale as you push up; exhale as you go down. Start with two of these and work up to however many you can do. It's a general body toner as well as an arm exercise.

Back Up

With your heels about one inch from the baseboard, back up to a wall and press the small of your back against the wall; hold for a count of ten; step away from the wall and try to walk that way. It'll improve posture and tighten those tummy muscles.

With your heels about six inches from the baseboard, back up to a wall; bend your knees, let your torso droop limply forward. Now, very slowly curl your backbone against the wall as you roll up to an upright position and raise your arms overhead. You should feel each vertebra in your back roll up against the wall. This is a relaxer as well as a back firmer and posture booster.

Here's a roll that doesn't put on pounds. Lying on the floor, with knees bent, clasp your knees and bring them to your chest as best you can; roll your head forward to touch your knees. Hold for a five count; unroll to original position. Repeat five times. This relaxes as well as stretches and tones.

To do this yoga backbend, sit on your heels, with your hands on your knees, then drop hands to your sides, touching your fingers to the floor. Slowly walk your hands back about twelve inches behind you, drop your head back as you raise your torso to do a backbend. Hold position about five seconds; reverse sequence of moves until you return to the original position. Repeat five times.

Bosom Buddies

Turn your coffee table into a bench press. (Make sure it's a sturdy one.) Lie on your coffee table with your feet flat on the floor and your head extended over the opposite edge. With your arms at your sides, bent slightly, grasp weights.

Be careful when choosing the weight that's right for you. You should start with a weight that you can easily use, then after a little while your body will tell you when to add more weight—*gradually*. Don't start with twenty-pound dumbbells! To firm and tone, use lighter weights and more repetitions; to build muscle, use heavy weights with fewer repeats. As you inhale, lift the weights up and back until your arms are stretched overhead and behind your head as far as you can toward the floor. Keep your lower back pressed into the table. Exhale as you return the weights to the original position. Work up to three sets of ten lifts.

In the same position as above, lift weights so that arms are straight up toward the ceiling. Inhale as you separate arms and lower the weights sideways toward the floor. Exhale as you lift the weights to their original position. Work up to three sets of ten lifts each.

Buttock Bumps and Fanny Firmers

Lie on the floor on your back, knees bent a hip width apart, feet flat on the floor. Keep your lower back flat on the floor. Tighten your buttock muscles as you raise your bottom, pressing your waistline into the floor; then lower and release. Repeat several times until your buttocks notice the command to tighten up.

In the same position as above, squeeze buttock muscles and rotate hips in a circle, first to the right and then to the left.

This exercise is for thighs and buttocks: kneel on the floor with your back straight and arms down, palms on thighs. Lean backward slowly, using your thigh muscles and keeping your spine straight. (If you don't keep your spine straight you'll be pulling on your back muscles instead of thighs.) Hold the backward lean for a ten count; return slowly to original position; repeat about eight times, allowing a breather between leans.

Face Lifters and Chin Uppers

Rest your chin on your fist, and try to open your mouth, pushing against your fist with your jaw. Repeat ten times.

Try this face firmer: tilt your head back, push your lower lip over your top lip; count to five, and then try to push your chin muscles up where your lip is for another five count. Repeat six times.

When you eat, choose foods that you have to chew hard—carrot sticks, celery, apples. In addition to working your jaw muscles, you'll be eating foods that are good for you. And did you know that celery and apples, like parsley, are natural breath fresheners?

Open your mouth and stick out your tongue, pointing the tip of your tongue as far toward the tip of your nose as you can. Do this twenty-five times and work up to more. You'll feel your neck tightening.

For Feet

Take a rolling pin or empty soft drink bottle and relax your feet by curling them and your toes around the curved surface. Some say this is also an arch strengthener.

Hip, Hip, Away

Lying on your stomach, with legs stretched out and pressed into the floor, first lift both legs as high as you can, making sure that you don't overarch the small of your back, then scissor-kick them, as if you were swimming, about twelve times. For especially good results, do this rapidly.

Lying on your stomach, with legs stretched out and pressed into the floor, alternate gentle kicks with each leg, pressing hip bones to the floor and tightening buttocks as you kick. Rock and roll a few times, and then follow by lifting and lowering both legs twice. Repeat the whole sequence of rock, roll, and lift about twelve times.

While you are on your hands and knees on the floor, bend your left knee, drawing it up to your chest while you drop your head; then kick up and back with your left leg as you lift your head high. Alternate legs and do this exercise at least ten times with each leg.

Legs

To strengthen your inner thigh and buttock muscles, lie on your side with your bottom knee bent slightly for balance. Prop your head up with your bottom-side arm, and place your top-side arm bent, hand on hip, fingers pointed toward your foot. Flex your foot so it's positioned as if you are walking, and then lift your top leg up toward the ceiling, as you keep it straight and aligned with the rest of your body. Your hips should be facing straight ahead. Hold for a count of six, and lower leg slowly. Repeat fifteen times on each side. If you add weights to your ankles you will get extra benefit.

Firm up inner thighs by lying on your back, with weights tied to your ankles. Lift your legs so that they are at right angles to your body, then open legs to a "V" or split position; close legs; repeat, doing three sets of ten splits each.

Firm up thigh fronts with this lift: with weights on your ankles, sit on a table or other surface that keeps your feet from touching the floor. Holding onto the table, lift your legs up so that they are level with the tabletop and completely straight; lower legs; repeat. *Remember your breathing.*

Firm up fronts of your thighs by walking up steps, two at a time, while you keep your hands clasped behind your back, speed skater style, pushing yourself up with toes on the lower step. Do this four times.

For toning hips and thighs, sit in a straight chair and cross your right leg over your left knee. Then put both hands, one on top of the other, on your right knee, and try to raise your right thigh and left heel from the floor as you push down with your hands. Cross left leg over right knee and repeat several times.

For shapely calves, stand on a thick book, your heels extending over the edge. Bracing yourself on a chair back, raise and lower your heels from tip toe to below top of the book level; repeat. Work up to three sets of ten lifts; then, to make it harder, repeat with one foot at a time. After you get used to this, you can also vary the exercise by alternating toes pointed in and toes pointed out on the lifts.

Office Toner

When you feel sluggish from sitting at your desk or on a plane, sit up straight and lift both feet from the floor at the same time, slowly stretching them up and out until they are level with the chair seat; hold them out in front of you for a ten count, and lower them to a ten count. Do this five times and just feel those muscles wake up and tone up.

For your upper arms and tummy, exhale all the air from your lungs and press your stomach in with your palms as you keep your elbows at right angles to your body. Inhale deeply through your nose and exhale through your mouth as you continue to press your stomach with your hands. You can do this one in an elevator —if you are alone.

For upper arms and bosom, fold your arms across your chest and as you clasp your hands on each opposite forearm, push against your arms with short, brisk movements. Try this one as you hang up your coat—people will think you're pushing up your sleeves and won't even know that you are a closet exerciser!

For your back muscles and hamstrings, pick up light objects (never heavy objects) from the floor by bending from the waist. But, of course, be careful about your rear view.

Tummy Tighteners

If you have the nerve and/or can be discreet, use standing time (while waiting for a bus or elevator) to pull in and hold those tummy muscles taut. Repeat ten times. Tuck buttocks under and hold, then release, about fifty times. Flex and relax calf muscles, about twenty-five times. Truck drivers may stare at you when they pass by your bus stop, but so what?

Now, lying on your back, feet and knees apart, feet flat on the floor, elbows pointed out, reach down and grasp the inner part of your thigh, putting your right hand on your right thigh and left hand on left thigh. Bend forward and hold this position for a seven count. Then slowly "walk" your hands down to your ankles, back up to your thighs. Release your hands and raise your arms straight up. Return to original position.

Lying on your back, with your knees bent, feet flat on the floor and arms straight at your sides, inhale as you tuck your chin into your chest, and stretch both arms straight forward; hold for a six count. Then exhale as you curl up, arms still stretched forward, as you stretch your left shoulder toward your right knee. Roll back down to the floor; turn your head from side to side, and then repeat this exercise with the other side of your body.

Lying on your tummy on the floor or in bed, with your upper body propped up on your elbows, slowly raise one leg as high as you can without bending your knee. Alternate legs and do each leg about eight or ten times.

To strengthen tummy and thighs, sit on floor (carpeted preferably) with your back straight and your arms extended in front of you. Pull your knees up to your chest, lifting your feet up from the floor. Still holding your feet up, first extend your legs forward, then pull them back to your chest, and extend again. This is a toughie, so don't try to do it more than once or twice right away; you can work up to as many repetitions as are comfortable, because this is a general toner as well as a special exercise for tummies and thighs.

Waist Away

While lying on the floor on your back, legs flat and arms outstretched at shoulder level, palms on the floor, bend your knees, lifting your feet about a foot from the floor. Hold legs in this position, knees together, as you roll side to side touching your outer thighs to the floor. Don't let your back arch. Repeat until your muscles notice.

Stand with your feet wide apart and your arms held over your head. Bend at the waist, to the right side, bringing your arms out in front as if you are reaching for something; then circle, in waist-bent position, to left. Repeat exercise five times to each side. This increases flexibility as it tones.

Stand with your feet apart and your arms overhead. Reach for the ceiling with your arms still overhead, lifting your rib cage, and bend first to one side and then the other. Repeat bends until you start to feel it in your muscles. Next, holding a book or other weight in your left hand, place your nonweighted right hand on your hip as you bend to the right. Change hands (and weight) and repeat ten more times.

Stand with your feet apart, knees slightly bent, and hands on your hips. Tighten tummy muscles and twist as far right as you can, then as far left. Do at least ten twists to each side. This is an easy beginning exercise for those who haven't twisted since the twist. As you get more limber, try putting your hands on your shoulders instead of hips, and then twist right and left for ten counts in either direction. Twist some more by holding your arms outstretched at shoulder height; twist alternate sides right to left for ten counts each side.

If you can't do a regular sit-up, try this: lying flat on the floor with legs together, put your hands behind your head, fingers interlaced. Then with heels on the floor, raise your head and shoulders until you can see your heels, pulling in your tummy. Lower head and shoulders; repeat ten times. Remember your breathing! Inhale on the rest, and exhale on the effort.

You can also try a bent-knee sit-up. Lie on your back, fingers behind your head and elbows up, with knees bent in, feet flat to the floor. In one move, sit up, bringing your elbows forward; roll back to flat position. Repeat and build up to at least twenty sit-ups.

Walk

Walk anywhere you possibly can; don't drive unless you have to. Walk at least twenty minutes—briskly, with heel-to-toe foot movements and arms swinging naturally—to get cardiovascular exercise, and you'll burn around 250 calories per hour. Walk instead of eating or taking a lazy nap. Park farther from your office door so you'll have to walk a bit, and walk to lunch when you can.

• POOL EXERCISE •

I think swimming is the most pleasant form of exercise—it's so easy to move in the water, it's cooling in the summer, and it's just plain fun. But, 'fess up—when you're in the water, you aren't swimming every single minute. In fact, I'll bet you spend half of your pool time just soaking and hanging on the edge.

Some people like to swim laps, but most private pools aren't long enough for lap swimming, and most public pools are too crowded to swim in. That's why I've collected some exercises that you can do in the pool to shape up in between soaking and resting.

Most swimming activities involve your back, so it's especially important to do some stretching warm-up exercises to avoid injury. The old arms-overhead-and-bend-from-the-waist-to-touch-your-toes routine is one good stretcher and warmer upper.

Here are a few of the pool exercises that I like to do. Hold a beach ball with both hands and force it under the water to your knees; hold it down for as long as you can to firm up arms, shoulders, and those important pectoral muscles that hold up your breasts.

Hang on the side of the pool and try to hold a beach ball under water pressed between your knees—great for the inner thighs!

Using your arms and shoulders to hang on the side of the pool, brace your back against the side of the pool and do some scissors-style leg crisscrosses, alternating right leg over left and left leg over right, until you feel like quitting. Build up the number *gradually*, or you'll get sore. In the same hanging position, try keeping one leg straight down and making giant circles with your other leg, turning your hips from side to side as you do the circles. Alternate legs, and repeat as often as you like.

Bounce on your toes, jumping high, keeping your feet together while you are in waist- or chest-deep water. This is not only an exercise, but one way to get used to the water if the temperature isn't exactly right.

Jog in place, keeping your arms in running position. I love doing this—there is no pounding on my knees and ankles as with real jogging.

Hanging on the pool's side, arms extended, raise your knees to your chin and then straighten your legs again. Repeat as often as you like. Then put your knees together and do some side-to-side twists, aiming your knees first to one shoulder and then the other. Repeat as often as you wish.

On your stomach, hands on the pool's side, float your body straight from the pool edge and, with legs together, circle your ankles, first in one direction then the opposite.

Face the pool edge, hang onto the side with your hands, and climb or walk up the side of the pool until your feet are near your hands; then walk back down. Repeat.

Hang poolside and kick in all directions.

Tread water.

Do any floor exercise you like while floating in the pool. They will be easier. Many people with arthritic joints can exercise in the pool more comfortably than on land because water, if you are in up to your neck, lessens gravity's pull by 90 percent. The feet and legs of a 130-pound person only have to support 13 pounds when that person is immersed in water. Wouldn't it be great to have a household scale that we could use under water! Then weighing yourself wouldn't be such a chore, would it?

Swimming laps is a great pool exercise, but make sure to increase the number of laps you do gradually. The way to get into swimming laps is to swim hard until you feel winded, ease off to a slower, easier stroke, like a side stroke, until you've recovered; then go at it full speed again. If you are in really poor condition, it's a good idea to swim a lap, get out of the water, and walk back, alternating swimming and walking for five or more laps. After you get in better shape, you can increase the total number of laps you swim.

• MEDITATION •

Meditation is a terrific stress reducer. It's also very effective in helping dieters avoid snacking and eating when they're not really hungry.

Try this: wear loose comfortable clothing. Turn down the lights. Find a quiet place, a comfortable chair. You can sit in a comfortable position or lie down on your back with legs comfortably apart and arms slightly away from your body. Close your eyes; forget your daily cares.

With eyes closed, imagine you're standing on a bridge looking at a slowly flowing black stream of water—the flow is moving away from you. Imagine that a bright light has appeared on the water, and it, too, is flowing away from you. As it gets farther away, it gets smaller but brighter, and it begins to spin. The light continues to go farther, get smaller, get brighter. And you are getting very calm and very relaxed.

Count to ten:

One—getting calm, getting relaxed, feeling good
Two—feeling dreamy
Three—feeling calmer, peaceful
Four—feeling so calm, feeling as if you're drifting
Five—drifting slowly, slowly
Six—drifting, feeling so relaxed
Seven—drifting, so nice
Eight—drifting

Nine—relax
Ten—relax

Stay in this relaxed state for about five minutes; then count backward from three to one.

Three—waking up, not tired, but feeling very relaxed
Two—waking up, feeling very refreshed, feeling very good, ready to do anything
One—open your eyes; move your arms and legs; feeling very good, very relaxed, very refreshed

If you can do this meditation twice daily for three weeks, you'll be able to do it automatically whenever you need to relax, and whenever you need to avoid eating.

Some people like to meditate just before bedtime; others like to do it after lunch. You need to find the time that is best for you so that you will keep it as a scheduled part of your daily life.

Here's another popular meditation technique:

Find a quiet place and settle down comfortably. Sit down for this one; you need to be physically comfortable so that you can give the following tense-up and relax messages to your body.

First, tense up as tight as you can, then completely relax each part of your body in the following order: toes, feet, ankles, calves, thighs, hands, arms, shoulders, and neck. When your neck muscles are relaxed, let your head fall forward. The tension is leaving your head, your face. Your temples feel relaxed, your eyelids feel relaxed, your jaw is loose, *you* are relaxed. You are totally, completely relaxed, from head to toe. Stay that way for five to twenty minutes.

Come out of your relaxation by slowly counting backward from ten to one; then open your eyes and "wake up." You will feel wonderfully refreshed.

One of my friends used this meditation technique to rest and keep her sanity when her five children were babies. She could turn her meditation on and her confusion off at will and swears that meditation got her so relaxed she even used it when she delivered her babies without or with minimal anesthesia.

Quickie Relaxer

For a quick relaxer, do a yoga shoulder stand or try propping your feet up on the wall as you lie on the floor.

When I am on the road and spending most of my time sitting on planes or in TV studios, or walking through miles of airport terminals (in heels no less!), this is what I do when I get to my hotel room. I rest my head on a pillow on the floor, put my feet as high as I possibly can on the wall or bed headboard and just let it all go. I've even been known (with no witnesses, thank heavens) to take phone calls in this position.

You can also get a fresh flow of blood to your brain by reclining on a slantboard. If you don't have one, use your ironing board. Rest with feet elevated (head down) for about fifteen minutes; longer if you have the time. It will wake up your brain and complexion and take the pressure off your legs, helping blood flow back to your heart.

· EXERCISING WITH MACHINES ·

Warm up before you exercise on machines and get instruction on their proper use so that you don't damage the very muscles you are trying to tone!

Breathing is key when exercising with machines. Remember to exhale when you're pushing or pulling weights; don't try to hold your breath. If you can't figure out when to inhale and when to exhale, just breathe normally; you can't go wrong with that. But however you do it, please breathe!

Don't overdo, or start with weights beyond your lifting capacity. Gradually build up to heavier weights, and always do the lift smoothly—avoid jerky movements that might hurt you.

When your routine is over, cool down for five or ten minutes by walking, running, biking or stretching, just as you did when you warmed up.

If you frequently feel pain when doing certain workouts, and you have followed the directions to increase gradually and are lifting smoothly, you may be doing the workout incorrectly. Find someone at a health club or "Y" to give you advice. Pain is not your goal; and if your workout is unpleasant, you'll soon quit.

· EXERCISE FACT AND FANCY ·

Breathing

Myth: establishing an inhale-and-exhale breathing pattern for each exercise you do is an absolute must.

Fact: whatever the exercise, weight lifting and other strengthening exercises will be easier and more effective if, as I've mentioned, you exhale on the lift and inhale on the let down part of the exercise. Although you may feel silly at first, it also helps if you make some sort of sound as you exhale. This is important. Trying to lift and inhale at once may hike up your blood pressure dangerously.

When you are jogging, swimming, biking, or doing aerobic dance or any other endurance-type exercise, the trick is not a trick at all —breathe naturally.

Cold Weather

Myth: if you jog, hang up your shoes in winter. Running will get you overheated and make you sick.

Fact: proper dressing for winter-weather exercising will keep you comfortable. Figure out by trial and error how much clothing you'll need. The rule of thumb: if you feel warm when you start out, you're probably overdressed. Layers are a good idea because you can peel them off and put them back on as your comfort zones change. Since most of your body heat is lost through your head, neck, and extremities, you need to wear a cap and, in colder weather, a turtleneck shirt, mittens or gloves, and warm socks. It's important to keep your feet dry. In icy conditions, wear shoes that provide good traction so that you don't slip.

If you begin feeling as if you are cooling down rapidly, go indoors, even if it means cutting your run short. If perspiration-damp clothing starts to cool, you can become hypothermic (develop low body temperature).

On windy days, start running into the wind when you have more energy and then you'll have the wind at your back when you are finishing your run and energy is lower. Sounds like an Irish or balloonist's blessing—may the wind be always at your back!

Daily Exercise

Myth: if you can't exercise every day, it's not worth exercising at all.

Fact: if you can exercise only one or two days a week for at least thirty minutes, it's worth the effort. If three days a week is your minimum goal, you will get the health benefits you need—loss of fat, more efficient heart action, lower blood pressure and pulse rate. Of course, if you exercise every day, you'll get maximum benefits.

Energy

Myth: because exercise is tiring, you shouldn't exercise unless you feel energetic.

Fact: almost any exercise will make you feel more energetic, in addition to reducing the stress that drags you down. I've found several studies that show even those who are overweight and under stress are healthier and feel more energetic if they follow a regular exercise program. The best rule you can follow is: never go more than twenty-four hours without some sort of exercise, even if it's only a few stretches, a brisk walk, or a few sit-ups.

Equipment

Myth: exercise equipment has to be fancy and expensive.

Fact: broomsticks or canes are good aids for a variety of posture exercises.

You can sew four heavy towels together for use as an exercise mat or, when the middle is worn, cut up a blanket's four corners and stick them together to make a mat.

Weights can be made with household discards. For example, fill strong plastic bags or double bags with two and a half or five pounds each of sand, buckshot, or cat box gravel. (Two and a half and five pounds are the most common weights for exercising.) Close the bags with a twistie or string and place each one inside an old sock, tying the socks shut with a string. You can also tie two socks together. You'll have either two lighter weights or, if you tie the socks together, one heavier one for exercising.

Socks filled with one or two pounds of sand, litter, or buckshot, can also substitute for ankle and wrist weights, to wear when you walk or run. Old terry tube socks can be easily pinned to wrap around ankles or wrists and, best of all, they'll be colorful and economical.

Weights for lifting can be made by filling handled milk, vinegar, or bleach plastic jugs (wash out first, of course), with sand, litter, or gravel to the weight you want. One of my friends has taped together four (one-pound) iron railroad spikes (two pounds each) that she found in the country to use for a pair of exercise weights.

And don't forget canned food. It's already weighed; just don't drop them; bacteria can get into cans that are dented at the seam.

Use your imagination for exercise equipment *before* you use your wallet or checkbook.

Feet

Myth: you need special shoes for exercise.

Fact: it depends on your workout choice. Go barefoot or wear stirrup tights when you are bending and stretching and you'll exercise your toes more and strengthen your feet.

You do need proper shoes for jogging or walking. They should fit properly, cup the heel to prevent shock, and cushion your entire foot; some people prefer the heel area to be twice as thick as the sole of a running shoe. Notice that the treads on the bottom are for specific sports and give you the kind of traction you need for outdoor asphalt or gravel, tennis or handball courts, and so forth.

The box that good sport shoes come in will state the use they're designed for.

Don't buy for looks; buy for action and the activity for which you'll wear the shoes. Some of the better brands have special arch supports for feet that turn in and for other foot problems, too.

Don't just grab the first pair you try on. Read the labels on shoes just as you do on foods.

If your shoes fit, and you still get blisters on your toes, it may be due to lifting your toes as you run and rubbing them on the top of your shoe. Try putting petroleum jelly on your toes or taping them to reduce the friction between your toes and shoe tops. You can also find sleeve-type bandages and foam protectors at the drug store. Make sure your shoes are big enough.

Flexing Your Muscles

Myth: it's okay to regularly stop halfway through a strengthening or stretching exercise if you want to get your session over in a hurry.

Fact: if you regularly stop short on a strengthening or stretching exercise, you won't get the full benefit and may actually lose some of the flexibility and strength you already have. Of course, this doesn't mean that you should do each new exercise to the maximum on the first day. The idea is to work up gradually to the maximum of an exercise and maintain that level of endurance.

Huff and Puff

Myth: if you can talk while exercising, you aren't working out hard enough. You should be huffing and puffing and rendered speechless.

Fact: when you are huffing and puffing and exhausting yourself, you probably are working too hard and won't be able to work out long enough to do yourself any good. When you are doing an aerobic/endurance exercise, you should be working at a level that enables you to just barely talk or sing.

Injuries

Myth: if it ain't broke, don't fix it.

Fact: don't ignore *any* injury. Ice, rest, wrap, and raise it, as needed.

Unless you have a fracture or injury severe enough to call for a physician's care, you can give yourself some tender loving care at home.

• *Ice:* apply ice to the painful area for twenty minutes, four times a day for three days.

• *Rest:* rest for a few days to allow healing, then rebuild strength to former level, but do so gradually. If you can't wait to continue exercising, try a workout that does not involve the injured part of your body.

• *Wrap:* wrap an injured wrist, ankle, or other part of the body with an elastic bandage, but don't wrap so tightly that you cut off circulation to any part of your body, and don't sleep with a bandage on.

• *Raise:* keep an injured foot or leg propped up whenever possible to help circulation go back to your heart. You'll have less swelling.

If you have chronic pain or frequently injure the same area, get professional medical help to determine how badly you've hurt yourself. Ask your exercise therapist or instructor if you are doing the exercise properly.

Leg Warmers

Myth: leg warmers are only a silly fashion fad.

Fact: leg warmers keep calf and thigh muscles warm and relaxed so they won't cramp up. Wear them during your warmup and throughout exercise/dance routines. You can make your own with old knee-high tube socks that have become toeless, or by cutting the sleeves from an old sweater that has lost its body—like the one that went through the dryer and became so short it bared your midriff. What you need is something that will keep your calf muscles cozy without cutting off circulation.

Massage

Myth: if you can afford massages, you don't have to exercise because they knead away fat.

Fact: because it increases circulation throughout the body, massage helps you get rid of excess water weight. Some people believe massage helps break down fatty tissues so the body can more easily dispose of them. But most of these same people believe that exercise complements massage by firming up your muscles. Everyone I know who gets massages says they are wonderful relaxers, and that includes me. But they should not be a substitute for exercise.

Numbers

Myth: if doing twenty-five sit-ups or any other calisthenic exercise is good, pushing yourself to fifty or one hundred is better.

Fact: train, don't strain, is the advice from the experts. When you are tired, you are likely to get sloppy about doing an exercise properly. For example, if you push yourself to do too many push-ups, instead of using your arm, shoulder, and chest muscles to pull your body up, you may begin to incorrectly arch your back and use your whole body to push up. The result will be a strained back instead of a firmer tummy. If you hurt yourself often enough doing exercises incorrectly, you'll soon quit. Who wants to keep doing something that's painful?

Quit when you begin to feel tired and notice you are cheating. Aside from avoiding injury, repeating an exercise incorrectly can become a bad habit, and you are trying to develop good habits for your body.

Pain

Myth: if it doesn't hurt, it's not doing much good. Work out until you feel pain. Muscles should really burn if you are working out properly.

Fact: there is a difference between muscles burning with pain and muscles feeling warm tension sensations. The heat felt while you are working your muscles hard enough is caused partly by a buildup of lactic acid in your muscles, which occurs normally during bursts of energy use.

Stop before you feel true pain and remember that a sudden sharp pain can mean injury. If a particular exercise always causes you to say ouch, you may not be doing it correctly or it may not be right for you.

Plastic Warmup Suits

Myth: plastic or rubber warmup suits are great for getting rid of fat fast. Zip up and zip along to sweat it all off.

Fact: rubber or plastic warmups dehydrate your body and deprive your skin of oxygen; avoid them. Better wear nylon, cotton, or terry warmups, and then only when you need them in an exercise room that is overly air-conditioned or outdoors in cold weather. The idea is to warm up from the inside out by exercising and, after vigorous exercising, let your body cool down naturally. Then put on a warmup suit if you need one to avoid getting chilled.

Speed

Myth: faster is better; do your exercises as fast as your body possibly can and, if you jog, do it in fourth gear, no matter what.

Fact: jogging is not racing; it's not the speed but the amount of time that you keep moving that counts. When you do other exercises, speeding them up usually causes you to use the wrong muscles and thus strain them or others. For example, when you do warmup stretches, you need to do them slowly. If your movements are swift and jerky, muscles will contract to protect themselves, and if you then stretch those contracted muscles, the result is pain and injury. Whatever the stretch, ease your way into it and then hold it about thirty seconds.

Timing of Exercise

Myth: you'll get the same benefits doing ten minutes of aerobic exercise three times a day as you will get if you do one session a day for at least thirty minutes.

Fact: thirty minutes should be your goal, but you need to work up to it *slowly*. Here's what happens when you exercise: first your body starts burning carbohydrates, then gradually it switches to burning fats. At about the twenty-minute point, you probably are burning about half fat and half carbohydrates; at about thirty minutes you are burning more fat than carbohydrates for fuel, which is what you want to do.

Don't be discouraged if you can't do thirty minutes on the first few tries at aerobic exercise, or if the first ten or fifteen minutes seem difficult. Your body adjusts to metabolic changes after the first fifteen to twenty minutes and, trust me, the exercise will get easier for you.

Yoga

Myth: yoga is only for people who have a guru to help them chant mantras. It calls for standing on your head or tying yourself up into knots.

Fact: not *all* yoga routines call for standing on your head or twisting into knots. Yoga is growing in popularity because it improves concentration, relieves stress, and enables you to gain strength and flexibility without working up a sweat or causing injury.

Those who practice yoga say that it clears the mind as it clears the body and energizes in a way few other activities do. It does—at least for me.

Like everyone else I know, I tried all kinds of exercise regimens, but finally settled on the exercise routine that works for me, just as you should. No exercise program is worth a pound of sweat if you don't stick with it and enjoy it. I have tried running (boring and bad for my knees), calisthenics (also boring). Finally I found yoga. Now I faithfully do a combination of yoga, stretching, and deep-breathing exercises. Then I follow the yoga with a cardiovascular workout of jumping on a minitrampoline. For fun, I add some Heloise dance and jazz movements. Since I travel a great deal, I can't take my tramp with me, but I can take my yoga routines wherever I go.

Chapter 11

HEALTH PROBLEMS

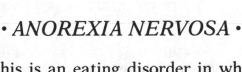 **· *ANOREXIA NERVOSA* ·**

his is an eating disorder in which victims, usually female (90-95 percent), of all socio-economic levels, starve themselves in an attempt to reach perfection and control over their lives. About 6 percent of victims die. Symptoms include abnormal weight loss; eating only tiny amounts; abuse of laxatives, diuretics, emetics, or diet pills; vomiting; denying hunger; compulsive exercise; depression; seeing oneself as fat although very thin; preoccupation with food, calories, and diet; menstrual irregularity or absence of periods.

The most effective preventive measure is psychological counseling. Self-help groups such as ANAD (Anorexia Nervosa and Associated Disorders Inc.), Box 271, Highland Park, IL 60035 can help. ANAD refers you to local groups and therapists. Send $1 for postage and handling for information packet. (Also for bulimics.)

The method of treatment for anorexia nervosa is behavior modification for healthy eating habits.

· *BACK PAIN* ·

Some causes of back pain are tension, injury, poor muscle tone in abdomen , and poor posture. It affects many, especially those people in their forties who don't exercise.

Preventive measures include stress management, exercising abdominal muscles with sit-ups, etc.

Treatment often includes weight control through diet.

· *BIRTH CONTROL RISKS* ·

Some problems commonly associated with birth control are heart disease risks for women over thirty-five, and overweight.

The use of low-risk birth-control pills containing twenty to fifty millionths of a gram of estrogen plus low-potency progestin can help avoid these risks. Also recommended are weight control and refraining from smoking.

· *BRITTLE BONES (OSTEOPOROSIS)* ·

Some causes of osteoporosis are not enough exercise, calcium, and/or vitamin D; too much protein or meat in diet; smoking. Most susceptible are petite, thin women in the sixty-plus age group.

Preventive measures include daily exercise, such as walking, jogging, biking, or rope jumping.

Vitamin D, and calcium (eight hundred to one thousand milligrams daily) can help in the treatment of osteoporosis. Also, avoid caffeine and cigarettes.

· *BULGING BELLY* ·

Some causes are overeating and weak abdominal muscles.

Test: lie down on back; place a ruler on your stomach with one end on your sternum, the other on your abdomen. If the abdominal end is higher than the sternum end, you have belly bulge.

Strengthen your muscles with sit-ups, walking, or running. Consciously tuck in tummy. Try isometrics.

Weight control with fiber-rich and low-fat foods is a necessary aspect of treatment of this problem. Some people should avoid salt.

• *BULIMIA* •

Indications of bulimia are binging, followed by purging by either inducing vomiting or taking laxatives to avoid weight gain. Laxative abuse leads to diarrhea, fluid loss, and chronic bowel dysfunction.

Psychological counseling is the recommended treatment. (See ANAD information under ANOREXIA NERVOSA.) Behavior modification for healthy eating habits is also part of the treatment.

• *CANCER* •

Research continues on this disease, but the best preventive measure is early detection. A few tips: fiber in your diet may prevent colon cancer. Avoid smoking. Protect your skin from sun exposure.

• *BAD POSTURE* •

Some typical forms of bad posture are slouching, and habitually keeping your arms folded across your chest. Tension can be a cause of posture problems.

Try yoga; isometric exercises; exercises for upper body; shoulder and neck massage. And learn to deal with stress.

Calcium will help keep bones healthy.

• *GUM DISEASE* •

This includes recession, bleeding, tooth decay, bone and tooth loss.

Some causes are poor mouth hygiene; brushing your teeth side-to-side too hard; too much junk food and sugar; lack of calcium. Gum disease often shows up when you're in your thirties.

Treatment includes, proper brushing up and down with a soft, multitufted brush; regular flossing to remove plaque; avoiding too much sugar.

A good diet, including at least 1,110 milligrams calcium daily, vitamin C foods, whole grains, greens, and vegetable proteins, will also help prevent gum disease.

• *HAIR (thinning, loss)* •

Some common causes are bleaching, perms, excess brushing, exposure to wind and sun, tight ponytails or braids, illness, hormonal changes, crash diets, stress, and heredity.

Some preventive measures are mild shampoos, cool drying, untangling hair with a wide-tooth comb, gentle brushing, avoiding hot combs and rollers, and the proper choice of ancestors.

A nutritious diet for this problem includes B vitamins, zinc, iron, vitamin E; low-fat, low-sugar, low-salt foods.

• *HIGH BLOOD PRESSURE* •

Some causes are stress, overweight, excess salt, and inadequate exercise.

Yoga, meditation, stress control, weight control, a regular exercise program, and avoiding salt will all help. And eat fruits and vegetables to get potassium; beware of salt-containing processed foods; get adequate calcium; use polyunsaturated oils and margarines.

• *HIGH CHOLESTEROL* •

Cardiovascular diseases such as atherosclerosis (hardening of the arteries) result from fatty deposits on the artery walls and lead to heart attacks and strokes. Too much saturated fat in diet, overweight, inadequate exercise, and smoking are some causes.

Learn to manage your diet for weight loss and maintenance; maintain a regular exercise program; don't smoke. Eat more fish, poultry, and fruits and vegetables and less red meat and dairy food; avoid saturated fats. Recent study shows eating several apples daily lowers cholesterol levels.

• *INJURIES FROM EXERCISE* •

Some causes of injuries are not warming up or stretching; an abrupt increase in activity; improper equipment or instruction.

To prevent injury, ease into stretching; and don't force it. Weight lifters should increase weights gradually, resting muscles every other day. Wog (walk-jog) before starting a full jogging program. Warm up and warm down for five minutes each before and after strenuous exercise. It takes at least three weeks for your body to adjust to new levels of exercise, so increase activity gradually. Wear shoes and clothing to match activity.

Apply cold compresses or ice immediately after an injury for the first few hours. Later, heat will relieve pain and hasten healing.

Good general nutrition is always a sensible preventive measure.

• *INSOMNIA* •

This is characterized by an inability to fall asleep, daytime drowsiness, irritibility, and restlessness.

To treat insomnia establish a pleasant bedtime routine and regular sleep schedule; avoid alcohol, caffeine, smoking, naps; avoid staying in bed too long, expecting more sleep hours than you need. Do relaxing exercises, but avoid strenuous exercise at bedtime.

Don't eat heavy meals at bedtime; but warm milk may help sleepiness.

• *JOGGER'S NIPPLES* •
(and other irritations of skin from sports)

Sore, tender, chafed nipples (or other skin areas) are often a result of exercise. To prevent them, cover nipples with petroleum jelly or an adhesive bandage when running; wear a sports bra and soft, textured T-shirts. In other areas, wear cotton undergarments, sew padding to protect knees or derrière (when biking); use moleskin to prevent blisters from your racquetball handle. For foot blisters and corns, get properly fitted shoes; wear terry socks.

· *LOSS OF MUSCLE AND STRENGTH* ·

This is caused by inadequate exercise and fitness. Regular exercise, such as vigorous walking, jogging, or swimming, will remedy the problem. Also follow rules of general good nutrition.

· *LUNG CAPACITY DECLINE (breathlessness)* ·

This shows up around age thirty. The decline is caused by inactivity. At least twenty to thirty minutes of aerobic exercise no less than three times weekly (even better, five times a week) is the answer. Try vigorous walking, jogging, swimming, biking, or dancing. Also, of course, follow rules of good nutrition.

· *OVERWEIGHT* ·

Tests: is there an inch of fat to pinch at your waist or right over your shoulder blades? Wrap a belt around your rib cage; try to slip it down past your waist without making it bigger; if it doesn't pass, it's time to lose weight.

Determine your ideal weight with this formula from the Dallas Aerobic Center: height (in inches) times 3.5, minus 108, equals weight. Large-boned women (wrist measures more than six and a half inches) can add 10 percent. For example, a large-boned woman, five foot, four inches tall, should weigh: 64 X 3.5 − 108 = 116 + 11.6 (10 percent of 116) = 127.6 pounds.

Change your life-style and eating habits to take in fewer calories and exercise more. Use other hints in this book as well.

· *SKIN (dry, wrinkled, brown spots)* ·

Causes of such skin problems include: too much sun, not enough moisture, harsh soaps and other products.

To treat, use sunblocks and moisturizers; protect your face with a hat and your hands with rubber gloves. Follow good general health practices and exercise.

Good general nutrition is an absolute necessity. Especially important are green, yellow, and orange vitamin A veggies; B-6, contained in brewer's yeast, whole grains, and poultry; polyunsaturated oil (about two tablespoons daily).

• *SWIMMER'S EAR* •

This is an earache, caused by irritations of the inner ear from pool or beach water.

Use earplugs. If store-bought ones are uncomfortable, make some out of cotton balls coated with petroleum jelly. Dry your ears with a few drops of alcohol mixed with vinegar dropped into the ear after swimming.

• *VARICOSE VEINS* •

They usually are caused by overweight, pregnancy, constipation, or heredity.

Exercise, such as walking and jogging, are good preventive measures. Also, avoid clothing that cuts circulation to legs, and try support or elastic stockings.

To prevent constipation, one of the causes of varicose veins, eat plenty of fiber, fruits, grains, and vegetables.

Chapter 12

YOUR BREASTS

W hatever their age, there are few women who can truthfully say that at one time or another in their lives they haven't tried to make their breasts shaplier, firmer, smaller, or larger. That trying may have involved everything from stuffing a training bra with facial tissues and socks to putting a bra in the freezer in the hope that stiffer would look fuller.

Breasts have no muscles. Rather, they are comprised of fibrous, connective, and fatty tissue. No exercise can make them bigger, but since they are supported by the pectorals, firm pectorals can make breasts appear bigger. Other support comes from a properly fitted bra.

· TO BRA OR NOT TO BRA ·

It's generally agreed that anyone larger than an A cup needs a bra to prevent breast tissue from sagging prematurely. There is a test you might try: put a pencil under your breast; if it falls, you don't need a bra; if your breast holds the pencil in place, it is too large to go braless without damaging tender tissue and causing stretch marks.

If your bra is not properly fitted, or does not adequately support your breasts, it's the same as not wearing one at all. A too loose bra allows stretching of ligaments and skin; a too tight bra inhibits breathing and because it has a "crutch effect," weakens those supporting pectorals.

• SPORTS BRA •

A sports bra is a must if you jog regularly. It should be made from perspiration-absorbing cotton and be mostly nonelastic so that it will survive frequent launderings. As mentioned earlier, sore nipples are a problem for some women who jog. You can alleviate some of the distress by wearing a proper bra; or you can put Band-Aids over your nipples or petroleum jelly on them to prevent soreness caused by friction.

• POSTURE •

Poor posture will help gravity pull harder on breasts and cause them to sag more than normal. Developing strong back muscles for good posture is an absolute must for large-breasted women. Any exercise that tones the back and arms will also tone the pectorals and give you firmer breasts. Shape is really determined by heredity, but good posture can make breasts look younger and perkier.

• PLASTIC SURGERY •

Plastic surgery can enlarge breasts. New polyurethane coatings on the implants prevent hard scar tissue from growing over the implant, so breasts no longer become hard, as was the case some years ago.

Breast-reduction surgery is more complicated than implanting breasts. Choose your surgeon carefully. (Refer to Chapter 12, "Cosmetic Surgery and Other Options.")

Reconstruction of breasts after a mastectomy is almost routine these days and is often done as soon as possible after the surgery, if no other treatments will be given.

• MEDICAL PROBLEMS •

It has been estimated that 90 percent of all women have problems with swelling, tenderness, fibrous tissue, thickening, or cysts at some time during their lives, but that these conditions should not be considered abnormal and should not be sources of worry.

The term "fibrocystic disease" is used, but women need to know that having fibrocystic breasts doesn't necessarily mean that you will get cancer.

An estimated one in eleven American women do have to deal with breast cancer in their lifetimes. The good news is that radical mastectomies (removal of the entire breast and surrounding tissue) are not performed as often as in the past. Instead, lumpectomies (removal of the tumor) with radiation therapy are more common.

The key is to discover the tumor in its first stages so that less tissue is involved. It is estimated that 95 percent of all breast lumps are found by women examining themselves.

Important: should you discover a lump, see your physician immediately. Be sure to get a clear explanation of all the treatment options available to you. You have the right to know exactly what will be done to your body.

Don't panic. Seek emotional support as well as medical help. Your doctor should be able to refer you to local support groups and counseling.

• SELF-EXAM •

All women twenty and older should regularly examine their breasts to note changes, lumps, or other irregularities as soon as they occur. You are the one who best can spot changes. This is most easily done in the shower while you are wet and soapy. Warning signs include a lump in the breast or under the arm, thickening, swelling, or distortion of the breast, pain or tenderness, irritation or dimpling of the breast skin, nipple discharge, retraction (going in), or scaliness. Any change that persists for more than a few weeks should be reported to a physician.

Eating foods lower in fat and higher in fiber may have a role in cancer prevention. (See "Diet Myths and Facts" in Chapter 10, "Shaping Up.")

Chapter 13

COSMETIC SURGERY AND OTHER OPTIONS

f you're unhappy about your complexion or have features you can't live with, there are medical procedures that can help. They include treatments to improve your skin as well as cosmetic surgery. What follows are brief descriptions of some of these procedures.

· CHEMICAL PEELS ·

Chemical peels can be performed in a dermatologist's or plastic surgeon's office or in the hospital. In general, this method works better for light, thin skin than dark, oily skin. It's especially good for removing fine facial wrinkles, crow's feet, and lines above the lip. Afterward you probably won't want to appear in public for a week to ten days, and depending on your skin, you may have a pink glow for as long as six weeks. It won't be until about six months after your peel that you'll be able to see the final results (no swelling or pink tone). You can wear prescription makeup to cover the pink, but above all avoid sun—even *reflected* sunlight—for at least several weeks after the bandages have been removed. (Bandages are removed about a day or two after the peel.) Even a few seconds of sun exposure can cause changes in the pigmentation of your skin and ruin the results of the peel. Prescription sunblocks should be worn until your physician says they are not necessary.

What exactly is done in a peel? A chemical, such as phenol, is applied to the skin to peel off the top layers of the skin, revealing the smoother layer underneath.

This procedure can be uncomfortable and expensive, depending on how deep the peel. The cost runs from $1,000 to $2,000 and up.

• *DERMABRASION* •

Good for the same fine lines that the chemical peel works on, this procedure also works the best for light, thin skin. It costs about as much as a chemical peel and is usually performed in the doctor's office. First your skin is numbed with ethyl chloride or another local anesthetic, and then surface lines and wrinkles are removed with a rotating wire brush or medical sandpaper. When it heals, the skin forms a crusty surface, which it sheds in about a week. But your skin stays red and sensitive for several weeks afterward, so, again, avoid sunlight. Like chemical peeling, dermabrasion can scar or leave dents where the skin is peeled or planed too deeply.

• *INJECTIONS* •

Injections of silicone, or a blood-protein fibrin that is taken from your own blood (fibrin foam), or a purified bovine collagen (Zyderm), all simply puff out whatever wrinkles, lines, or scars, such as pits from acne, you're trying to remove. Results take two to three months, and injections are often done at three- or four-week intervals. The cost is $100 to $200 per treatment—expensive, but perhaps the best choice for people who don't yet need a surgical face-lift and simply want to "repair" lines. You may need several office visits to get all the lines filled in, and the bovine collagen may only have a temporary (one to three years) effect. Why? In time, it is absorbed by the body, whereas silicone is permanent. Liquid silicone has a bad reputation from its abuses in the breast implantations of the 1960s and 1970s. At this writing, silicone has not yet earned FDA approval. In fact, silicone injections have become controversial. One to 3 percent of patients are allergic to Zyderm, which at this writing is still being evaluated.

• *BLEPHAROPLASTY (EYELID REPAIR)* •

This type of surgery will take care of puffy, baggy eyes. The cost for eyelid repair runs from $1,500 to $3,000, and up. It is usually done under local or general anesthesia. For about two weeks afterward, there will be some discoloration around your eyes, and sometimes your eyeball will become discolored due to some bleeding. There may also be some fine-line scars on your upper eyelid and just below your eyelashes in the lower eyelid. These lines are barely visible. In general, eyelid surgery is a fairly straightforward procedure; rarely are there major complications.

• *RHYTIDECTOMY (FACE-LIFT)* •

Face-lifts start at about $3,500 to $5,000 and go up. In general, plastic surgery of this sort is not for people under forty. But occasionally an under-forty person will get a minilift. Sometimes just the eye repair will hold up for four or five years before a person will undergo the procedure for jowls, saggy cheeks, etc. A face-lift is done under local or general anesthesia, and is often combined with eyelid, forehead, and/or brow lift. For several weeks afterward, you won't look very good because of discoloration and puffiness; it's a good idea to allow at least three or four weeks before going back to your social or work life. For a few months afterward you will experience some numbness in the cheek and neck area. Watch for excessive bleeding in the early postsurgery period; it can slow healing if not treated and in rare cases cause nerve damage to face muscles.

• *CHIN AUGMENTATION* •

Chin augmentation usually improves your profile by lifting sagging jowls. In this procedure, a silicone implant is inserted either through the mouth or through an incision beneath your chin. Afterward, you may experience some numbness and swelling in the chin and lip area, but the recovery period is short. You can go back to your regular activities soon afterward, as long as you protect the area.

• *RHINOPLASTY* •

A nose job involves changing the shape of the cartilage and bone that forms your nose and is done under local or general anesthesia. For about a week afterward, you will probably have some packing in your nostrils and a splint around your nose, along with swelling and discoloration and black eyes, which may last up to two weeks. The complete healing process takes three or more months.

• *BREAST AUGMENTATION* •

According to plastic surgeons I spoke to, breast implants have become safe. They do not increase your chances for developing breast cancer, nor do they mask lumps in your breasts. You will, however, have scars around the implant areas, and some women develop more scars than others. (After a mastectomy, breast reconstruction is no longer considered "cosmetic" and is therefore generally covered by insurance.)

• *BREAST REDUCTION* •

This is one procedure that, though not considered a "cosmetic" operation, may be covered by insurance. You will have some scars and may experience numbness of the nipple and some of the skin below the breast area. In certain cases, there is a loss of tissue as well.

• *BREAST UPLIFT (MASTOPEXY)* •

The famous stripper Gypsy Rose Lee, when asked by a reporter if she still had the same things she always had now that she'd reached middle age, reportedly replied, "Sure. I still have what I always had, but everything's two inches lower."

If you really can't or don't want to deal with everything being a little bit lower, here's what a plastic surgeon can do for you. Mastopexy improves the contour of the breast. While you are under general anesthesia, the surgeon lifts the breast tissue on the chest wall and repositions the nipple and areola (area around the nipple). There will be scars beneath the breast, running from the crease below the breast to the areola.

• *TUMMY TUCK (ABDOMINOPLASTY)* •

This procedure may include repair of weakened abdominal muscles, as well as removal of excess and flabby skin on the abdomen and repositioning of the navel. You will usually have a bikini area scar and will probably have to stay in the hospital at least several days.

• *THIGH, BUTTOCK, OR ARM LIFTS* •

Removal of excess skin from these areas results in permanent scars. Be sure to discuss explicitly the effects of this procedure with your surgeon.

• *SUCTION-ASSISTED LIPECTOMY* •

Fatty deposits under the skin are removed by suction. However, dimpling of the skin and other healing problems can result. This procedure should not be used to make you slim; its purpose is to remove stubborn fatty deposits from areas that won't slim down, such as "saddlebags" or tummy sags. The procedure is relatively new in this country, so be sure to shop around for an experienced practitioner before making your decision.

Here is some good advice from my friend Tolbert S. Wilkinson, M.D., who is certified by the American Board of Plastic and Reconstructive Surgery.

If you are considering plastic surgery, your most important consideration is the doctor's skill and experience. Get recommendations from former patients (several, if possible), as well as from other doctors. After all, it's your face and your body, right? You don't want to spend the rest of your life looking in the mirror at a mistake.

Plastic surgery can make a positive change in your life. Although it won't make you look eighteen again, a face-lift can cut about five years off your age. Don't be afraid of or embarrassed about considering it.

The American Society of Plastic and Reconstructive Surgeons (ASPRS) operates a referral service from which you can get the names of three board-certified plastic surgeons in your area who perform whatever type of surgery you are considering. You can get this information by contacting: Mary Peterson, ASPRS, 233 North Michigan Ave., Suite 1900, Chicago IL 60601 (312-856-1834).

ASPRS doctors are certified by the American Board of Plastic Surgery and/or the Royal College of Physicians and Surgeons of Canada and/or the Corporation Professionelle des Medicins du Quebec.

Certification means that a plastic surgeon has spent at least five years after graduating from medical school in general surgery and plastic surgery training programs. After this training, the plastic surgeon must pass rigorous written and oral exams in order to get certification.

Other surgeons, with backgrounds in other medical specialties, may perform plastic surgery. But the ASPRS recommends that you find out about the credentials and background of any of these surgeons before you make your decision.

Not everyone is a good candidate for plastic surgery. Plastic surgeons consider several factors before accepting you as a patient. Make sure you understand exactly what is going to happen during and after surgery. Here are some questions you and your surgeon need to consider:

1. Do you have any health problems that might make surgery risky? The surgeon will tell you about the risks, hazards, and limitations of the particular type of surgery you're considering.
2. Is it realistic to expect that the part of your body that you want changed can actually be altered to your satisfaction by the procedure? The surgeon should explain the procedures with pictures and diagrams, offering the truth about what to expect

during and after surgery. Remember, there are no guarantees in surgery.

3. Are you emotionally suited to undergo this surgery? Or are you being influenced by well-meaning and possibly poorly informed friends or family members? You can't expect surgery to solve all your problems.

4. Do you recognize the limitations of the surgery you are considering? You may need a combination of procedures for certain results. For example, to reduce scarring you may need both dermabrasion *and* injections of collagen.

Chapter 14

CLOSETS:
BEHIND CLOSED
DOORS

f every time you open your closet door you get hit with an avalanche of shoes and hand-bags, it's time to organize.

Every six months—or better yet, at the change of each season—weed out and reorganize your closet. I find that this really saves time when I'm picking and choosing to get dressed or packed for a trip.

Start by packing up the clothing you know you will never wear. Don't forget those blouses and dresses that have been on hangers so long they have hanger dust lines on their shoulders. If you haven't worn it in a year, give it the old heave-ho. A local women's shelter or other organization will put it to good use. If you give never-worns to a worthy cause, you won't feel guilty about not saving them; you'll be helping someone else, and there's a bonus: they're a tax deduction!

Now, I know that there are certain things that you just can't let go—the dress you use as a fatness gauge (when it doesn't zip, you diet), or the one you were wearing when you met Him. Sentimentality need not mean clutter. Just hang those "memorials" in another closet—the one where you'll be hanging your off-season clothing once your closet is organized.

I don't think you should ever throw away any garment made from real wool, linen, or pure silk. Garments made from real, natural fibers can usually be altered to accommodate style and size changes. If you follow fashion, you know that some styles never change and some come back after a few years; so hold onto those garments made with classic materials!

• READY? SET! GO! LET'S ORGANIZE! •

Here are some tips for organizing your closet:

Divide to Conquer

Take all off-season clothing and "memorials" and put them in another closet.

Now, divide your clothing into categories. You can separate by coordinating colors; or by breaking down into office, home, play, and partying categories; or type of garment, such as skirts, blouses, vests, jackets. I divide my clothing by type and then color—and that includes accessories such as pantyhose, shoes, handbags, and scarves. I've even given pantyhose a subdivision: sheer and opaque!

You can separate the categories with a hanger covered with a cleaner's bag or you can use different-colored hangers to mark each group—much as they separate sizes on a department store rack. You can make cardboard or colored posterboard dividers modeled after the doughnut-style dividers some department stores use (Sorry dieters, that's the best description I can think of!)

While you are dividing your clothing, pull out buttonless blouses, skirts with taped hems, and slacks that have air-conditioned seams. If anything needs repairs, do it now so that you won't have to later, at the wrong time (like when you're dressed and ready to leave the house). If you don't sew, find a dry cleaner with a tailoring service, or a seamstress. The money you spend on having your mending done will at least put these garments back in circulation instead of in the back of your closet. While you're at it, take the dry cleanables in. Remember, a spot ignored may be a spot forever!

Keep Your Things in View

Have you ever noticed that you don't wear the things you can't see? When you start putting your clothes back into your closet take into account the fact that you're not likely to unzip bags or uncover boxes or rummage to the bottom of a drawer every morning.

Put shoes on racks, or remove the ends of shoe boxes so that you can see what's inside when they are stacked. You can also stash shoes or other small items in the paperboard nine-section divided boxes that are often on sale at dime stores. You can see your sweaters and T-shirts better if they are stacked on a closet shelf instead of in a drawer. And there's a bonus: this way they're less likely to get squashed. If you don't have enough shelves, try putting an old bookcase inside your closet beneath blouses and jackets.

Clear plastic storage boxes are great for shoes, scarves, sweaters, and such, but you can save money by using cartons with the ends cut off.

If you *must* cover a garment, use an old sheet or pillowcase—furs and leathers need to breathe and can be damaged by storage in plastic bags. When I store coats and other similar garments, I use the plastic cleaners bag, but cut it off about three or four inches below the shoulder. This keeps the dust off, but still lets you see the garment.

Decorate with It

If you are really short on space, why not use your colorful accessories to decorate your room? Necklaces, hats, scarves, and other accessories can be hung on peg boards, or with any of the hanging suggestions below so that they add color instead of just clutter to your life.

Baskets and old spice racks or lazy susans are among the many holders for your cosmetics or small accessories that can also personalize your room as decorator items. Think twice, too, about the odd wine glass or mug that doesn't match anything in the kitchen; it can be put to good use on your bureau to hold makeup brushes or change.

Hang It!

If it can hang, hang it. Even knit dresses and sweaters can hang on padded hangers. Hang knit or sweater dresses over the hanger from the waist. Padded hangers are expensive, but you can make your own: unwind the twisted neck of the hanger and thread the wire mid-width through four-inch-wide strips of nylon net, making a thick ruffle on all but the hook part of the hanger (in coordinating colors, if you like). Nylon-net ruffled hangers make especially good drip-dry hangers because air circulates through the nylon padding.

For a really neat padded hanger that looks as if it, and you, have a sense of humor, pad a wire hanger with old pantyhose. Just poke the hanger hook through the crotch of the panty and wrap each leg loosely around the hanger. Pull the panty over all this. The elastic in the waistband will hold the legs in place.

And if you don't have enough space for hangers, try hanging a chain from your closet ceiling—you'd be surprised at what can be hung on it. Hang your belts on it by color, and you'll never have to rummage around looking for the right one.

If you need an extra closet rod, try a spring-tension rod to make a two-tiered hanging area. Or just install a permanent second closet rod beneath the first. Another temporary solution is to attach a piece of wire or a strong cord to each end of the closet pole to form a loop. A hanger, hung on the rod with its "shoulders" pulled into a loop, works too. After you form a loop on each end of your closet rod, run a second rod through the loops. You can use an old broom handle for this "hanging" second rod.

To color coordinate closet rods and to make hangers slide on more easily, I cover my closet rods with plastic shower curtain rod covers. These plastic covers are often on sale or at discount stores and usually cost around a dollar.

Look for sales on multipant, skirt, and blouse hangers. These save lots of closet space, especially if you use them to store out-of-season clothing.

Go to the dime store and get the cheapest towel racks you can find. Attach them to the walls or door of the closet and you'll have handy pants hangers and/or a good place to loop belts, scarves, and shawls.

Cup hooks screwed into the wall or door will be an extra helping hand as you button those dresses and blouses onto their hangers *before* putting them on the closet rods.

If you put a rubber ball over a hang-up hook and then hang your jacket on it, your jacket won't get a funny-looking knob showing where the hook was. It won't slip off, either.

A slanted ceiling in an attic closet need not be a space waster. Just glue or nail clip-type clothespins on the ceiling, and use them to hold gloves, scarves, caps, or other small items that usually end up unmated after being stuffed in a drawer.

Look for decorator clothes stands at secondhand stores—or buy an over-the-door hanger. Use these to hold what you'll wear in the morning, or to air out what you've worn the day before. Just remember that it doesn't have to air *forever*. Also, use it to hang mending and clothing headed for the cleaners.

Dime-store metal tie racks on your closet wall or door can be used to hang up scarves, belts, necklaces or anything else that could spend its life tangled up in a drawer.

Those mesh, three-tiered hanging vegetable baskets don't have to stay in the kitchen—you can store all sorts of things (socks, hair rollers, etc.) in them in your closet or in a bedroom or bathroom corner.

When the paper tubes on wire hangers from the cleaners break, don't toss the whole hanger out, just the tube. Bend the ends up, and you'll have the perfect hook/hanger for sundresses, lingerie, scarves, belts, and the like. Regular hanger ends can also be bent into hook-enders for strapped garments.

Another way to keep sundress straps on a hanger is to wrap the hanger ends with rubber bands. Or you can hang them on a padded hanger.

If your clamp-type wooden pants hangers lose their grip, a strip of moleskin stuck on the insides will make them as good as new—maybe better.

Shelve It

If you're short of storage space for off-season clothes, fold them up and store them in large, heavy, plastic garbage bags. Toss a bar or two of unwrapped soap or a used fabric softener sheet into the bag so that your clothes will smell good when you take them out again. Seal the bags with a twistie or tape so your clothing won't host a party of winged or crawly creatures while it's hibernating. You can also put off-season clothing in a large trash can; make a tabletop cover with fabric or a large round tablecloth and not only get a place to store off-season clothing, but an extra lamp or end table.

An extra shelf is easy to add, even if you have no carpentry talent at all. Just put a board across bricks, cement blocks, wastebaskets (in which you've stored off-season foldables), or anything else that's square or rectangular and will hold a board.

You can make shoe shelves by using one-pound coffee cans (or other suitable cans) to brace up a board. Shoes fit nicely under the board, and you can stack cans and boards for more shoe-height shelves.

When you are shelving and stashing sweaters, slacks, or other garments, stuff tissue in the folds, or roll them to prevent fold-up creases.

· CLOSET MECHANICS ·

I don't know anyone who likes to wrestle with tangled hangers. First of all, if you move each empty hanger to the end of the rod after you remove the garment, you won't have to dig around when you want to hang it up again, or when you are taking clothes out of the dryer and need hangers pronto. When you fiddle around in the closet looking for empties, everything will get crushed.

One of my readers sent in this hint: when you have all your clothes out of the closet, take the closet rod (if it's wood) and make notches the same depth as hanger hooks. This will keep each hanger in place.

Or if you just want your hangers to slide better when you're moving them on the closet rod, apply some paste wax to the rod. Hangers will zip by. The colored plastic shower curtain rod covers mentioned earlier will also help your hangers slide back and forth, and you can use them to color-code sections or sides of the closet.

Do you have a light in your closet, but still grope around because you can't find the chain in the dark? Try attaching something you can hold on to, such as a fishing float. These come in cork or plastic; or, for a freebie, use plastic lemons or limes after you've used up the juice. The lemon is especially easy to see.

Can't stand the clutter of your closet shelves? Hang a shelf-length curtain over it; just use a spring-tension rod at the ceiling.

If you have to share a closet, divide the space evenly so that you can remain friends with your closet buddy. Either put up a marker of some sort in the middle (see separating clothing) or paint each half of the closet or closet rod a different color.

If you are desperate for more closet space, and if you have an alcove in your room, the alcove can be covered with a curtain or roll-up blind, and you can hang clothes either on a spring-tension rod (if one will fit), or on one of those portable clothing racks you find in catalogs and, of course, thrift shops. Even hooks on a peg board can hold clothing. When in need, use your imagination!

• *CLOSET CURES* •

An almost-aired-out room deodorizer will give up its last gasps of scent in a closet without causing you to gasp.

Cedar chips can be put in a nylon net bag or old nylon stocking to freshen a closet.

You'll have a sweeter-smelling closet if you open the windows, then open your closet doors a few hours each day or night and air them.

Air clothing before you put it back. Turn garments inside out to air, if you are one of those folks who really work up a sweat, or a "moist glow," if you are a woman who refuses to admit that she sweats. Some people say horses sweat, men perspire, and ladies glow. Call it as you see it, but whatever you call it, don't put clothes back into your closet until you freshen them with an airing.

I like to sprinkle baking soda on the floor of my closet and in my shoes and nonleather boots. I make my own deodorizer by filling a small jar with holes punched into its lid with cotton balls that I've sprinkled with oil of wintergreen or a favorite scent. You can also sprinkle a few drops of your favorite fragrance on the cotton.

In a small space, such as a drawer or cabinet, an opened empty perfume bottle uses up the absolute all of the perfume's fragrance for your pleasure. Storing soap in your closet and drawers is another good way to put fresh and pleasant smells into it. Years ago, I remember being told that soap stored without its wrappers becomes dryer and therefore lasts longer once it is put to use in water. Even soap wrappers can be used to provide the soap fragrance. You don't need to waste anything!

Mildew is a real problem for people who live in damp climates. If you have mildew in your closet, brush it out or vacuum it off the closet walls and floor, and any affected shoes, belts, or clothing. Air clothing or, if necessary, have it washed or dry-cleaned. Vacuum the closet until all mildew is gone, then throw away the bag if disposable, and clean off all attachments used so you won't be storing the mildew.

A mild alkaline solution, such as trisodium phosphate (from hardware stores) with warm water, or a bleach solution, can be used to scrub walls, etc. But test first to make sure the solution won't damage surfaces.

Once you get the mildew out of the closet, you can prevent it from growing back by sprinkling paradichlorobenzene moth crystals in the closet, or hanging bags of para crystals in the closet. *Caution:* the crystals can damage plastic buttons and ornaments. As always, you want to keep chemicals away from children or pets.

Make a homemade "demustifier" by filling a coffee can with charcoal briquettes. It will help ease the problem of damp closets. Punch holes in the lid, and keep the can on the floor. The larger the closet, the larger the can size.

In very damp climates, you may need to use special lamps or heaters to prevent mildew. *Caution:* you can cause a fire by using an ordinary lamp that gets overheated.

I keep my closet lights on all of the time. I think it's worth the few extra cents per month on the electric bill to protect my clothing and I've never had a mildew problem. If the thought bothers you, keep the light on just ten to fifteen hours a day or all night long.

Chapter 15

CLOTHES: CREATING THE RIGHT ILLUSION

*y*our wardrobe is, to a certain extent, a reflection of the unique you—your life-style, figure, personality—and, of course, the occasion. But there are some fashion tips that work most of the time for most people, no matter what's in style. Above all, it's important to keep in mind that what we see on those models is usually a bit extreme for us ordinary mortals.

So, try these dressing tips on for size.

· *TAKING OFF WEIGHT BY PUTTING ON THE RIGHT CLOTHING* ·

Vertical lines and dark or neutral colors can hide as much as five to eight extra pounds.

Longer jackets on suits and dresses hide a multitude of sins; short, waist-length jackets tend to make you look bulky.

Vertical patterns on prints force the eye to go up and down instead of side to side and all around. Avoid polka dots, geometric or checkerboard plaids.

Make vertical lines with accessories—a long strand of beads or pearls or long chains; a long, colorful scarf or tie, knotted at the bust line with ends draping down beyond your waistline, worn against a dark or neutral solid-colored dress.

Put the focus near your face; avoid drawing the eye of a beholder to any bodily bulges. Don't cut yourself in half, visually and physically, with bright-colored, tight belts or ones that wrap and tie, creating a bulky look. I wear narrow belts that blend in with the rest of the outfit. Straight-line dresses worn beltless flatter many women who carry weight in their midsections. Matching tops and bottoms give the illusion of longer, slimmer lines.

Hemlines are best kept at a medium length; too short will look skimpy and too long will make you look as if you are standing in a hole (especially if you are short).

Be realistic when you look in the mirror. Buying a size too small just because you can't face the reality of a larger size just means you end up looking like a stuffed sausage. Blouses that gap at the bust, pants that look as if you have been melted and poured into them, skirts with pockets that are perpetually open from tummy strain—none of these look good. Be objective. If you can't, bring along a friend—an honest one. Clothing that feels uncomfortable doesn't get worn, and that means you're wasting your money.

Buy quality. Well-made garments won't show stress and strain at the seams.

Avoid bulky-looking, thick woolen or mohair fabrics or delicate see-through filmy fabrics that show more than you want to show. Also, avoid big, outsize details such as huge, puffy sleeves or ruffles and bows.

If you are full-figured, shop in stores that specialize in garments and accessories for larger women. You'll find items proportioned for height and size so that you will get a better fit, not to mention a better selection of flattering styles for larger figures.

I have a friend who has been shopping in the petite department for years—since she lost her size-8 figure. She insists that size fourteen petite (the largest petite size) is perfectly proportioned to her five-foot, four-inch frame. It provides a better fit in the neckline and sleeve length as well as skirt length, but allows more room in the middle, where her extra weight has accumulated. So, I guess the moral is, don't be afraid to try specialty shops and departments if you don't fit into regular juniors or misses sizes. You don't have to tell anyone where you shop!

• DRESSING HINTS FOR THIN WOMEN •

But what about those lucky women who need a look that creates the illusion of added weight? Well, it's really hard for me to write this section—who doesn't envy the woman who can layer coat upon jacket upon sweater upon vest upon blouse or dress, and *still* not look like King Kong with a body shave and a human wardrobe? But, jealousy aside, my advice is to follow the reverse of the directions for looking slimmer. Wear horizontal lines, prints, plaids, and fabric textures that add weight. Ruffles, gathers, yolks, blousons, tucks, all flatter the thin figure.

If you are really bony, avoid the bare look and sleeveless tops. Disguise a thin neck and protruding collarbones with necklaces or chokers; upper-arm bracelets may be a good camouflage for thin arms. In general, skinny people, just like those who could afford to lose a few pounds, should avoid skin-hugging, slinky, clingy fabrics.

• BOSOM BUSTERS •

Just as most of us envy slim women, many of us envy women for whom bust-line darts in blouses and dresses actually have some significance. But, actually, having a large bust can be uncomfortable both physically and emotionally. Many large-busted women are continually embarrassed and annoyed by the attention their figures draw. Real people don't want to jiggle like a TV star, so the right bra is important. Large-busted women need good support and bras that minimize with soft shapes. Thanks to new fabrics and designs, the old-fashioned stiff harnesses are gone.

Big-busted women often try to hide their bosoms with a slouch, but the best camouflage is clothing. Avoid wearing sexy, clinging fabrics and fitted, figure-emphasizing garments to the workplace. Bright colors emphasize; deeper, darker colors disguise. Jackets with skirts or dresses are good bets, and try those that are unstructured and hang smoothly without hugging the waist. Any style that features a pinched-in waist will emphasize the bust line.

Women with extremely large breasts may need to lose weight or consider breast-reduction surgery.

• *LOOKING GROWN UP WHEN YOU'RE PETITE* •

Did you know that the National Center for Health Statistics has found that 55 percent of the women in the United States are five feet, four inches and shorter? That means that, at five feet, five inches, I'm taller than average—a fact that lifts my spirits, because my girl friends are all five feet, seven inches or taller and I've always felt short. More firms than ever before are making petite sizes, and so the selection for petites is much better than it was years ago, when petite women had to shop in the children's department. You'll still find bargains in sportswear there, but business and dress-up clothing need to be more womanly.

Being tiny can be a disadvantage in the business world, where "cute" doesn't really make an authoritative statement no matter *how* sharp you are. The advice from the experts to petite women is: get rid of frilly, little-girl mannerisms and such clothing touches as ruffles, cap sleeves, Peter Pan collars, sailor dresses, pastel colors and prints, shoes with flower decorations at the toe. Strive for a classic look: tops and bottoms of the same color family will make you look taller; wear belts that blend in with your outfit so that you don't cut your height; avoid contrasting colors and prints at skirt hemlines; coordinate your look so that accents are at your face, with lighter and brighter colors at the top; coordinate stockings with your dress and shoes so that the impression of a longer line is given, wearing light stockings with light outfits and dark stockings with dark outfits. Ordinarily, stockings are a shade lighter than your shoes. Small women get a longer look with pumps than they do with strapped shoes—these cut your feet off at the ankle. Small women need to wear makeup and hairstyles that avoid the pixie look. But of course, when you want to feel like a pixie at home or for play, wear and enjoy pastel-colored frills if you like them. Remember the golden rule: dress for the occasion.

If you keep your weight down, and if you can find clothing in the right proportions, you can wear some of the exotic looks enjoyed by those people who tower over you. But check proportions and try to keep the look simple and uncluttered.

• *TALL MEANS NEVER HAVING TO SLOUCH* •

But tall does mean searching for slacks that don't stop at mid-calf and skirts that aren't forever mini. Keep track of brands of clothing that fit—and flatter—and you'll save a lot of time.

Designer clothing is made for you; it fits all those glamorous models, doesn't it? Also made for you are textured fabrics such as mohair, cashmere, and tweeds.

If you are long-legged, you can blouse big tops to get better proportions; if you are long-waisted, you can wear exotic wide belts.

Avoid teeny, tiny prints, jewelry, and details on clothing; they are for teeny, tiny folk. You might also avoid two-piece dresses, which may give everyone a bird's-eye view of your midriff whenever they separate as you move your arms. Always try on such garments to be sure they are long enough. In fact, it's a good idea to always try on *anything* you buy.

If you find a blouse on sale that is definitely you, but has sleeves too short to reach your wrists, see if you can roll the sleeves up for a casual look.

• *LOOKS THAT MEAN BUSINESS* •

When you start assembling a professional wardrobe, look for power colors—dark, strong, and rich (rather than light, subdued, and bright)—simple lines, and quality. Quality means mostly natural fabrics and nontrendy accessories, including classic handbags, briefcases, and shoes.

Classic and businesslike need not mean dull and boring. The business suit "dress-for-success" uniform has given way to a more individualized look, but still, overdone is not done. If you feel as if you look your best and are appropriately dressed, you will feel confident enough to succeed in anything, whether it's a dress or a suit.

Perhaps uncluttered is the best recommendation for a business look: uncluttered design, fabric, print, accessories, hair, makeup. The clue is to look at the way women above and below your position in your company dress and adapt that look to your own style. For example, if suits are it with your female bosses, but you have broad shoulders and look hefty in them, a sweater-jacket may be the way to fit in.

If you live in jeans but want to look right at the company picnic, try wearing good-quality slacks and an interesting top. Some fashion experts warn that it's not a good idea to get really exotic when you go to company social events; you don't want people to start wondering just who you are deep inside, do you?

To dress well for work, most fashion experts agree that a mix-and-match wardrobe of two-piece dresses, suits, and/or separates will give you the most mileage for the minimum cost. (See Chapter 15, "Wardrobe Planning: Making More of Less.")

• *LOOKS THAT HAVE NO BUSINESS AT ALL* •

No matter how carefully you put yourself together for any workday occasion, you'll lose points if you wear:

• A blouse with a collar so high or a neckline so low that you are forever tugging at it

• A scarf tied in some complicated fashion that needs constant adjusting

• A suit or dress with a loose or missing button

• Jangling jewelry, especially bracelets—a real no-no when you're reading your report to an assemblage of company VIPs

• A bra or slip strap that plays peek-a-boo at your neckline or a bra or panty outline that's not invisible

• Anything that has spots anywhere, or a ripped hemline

• Scuffed, shineless shoes or shoes with heels that obviously need a lift or resoling

• Sling-back pumps that tell workers in the next building you are clacking your way along the hall

• Heels so spiky and needle-thin they become impaled in rugs and/or sidewalk gratings, rendering you immobile

• Pantyhose with runs

• Reinforced toes on pantyhose that peep out of open-toe shoes (one of my pet Heloise hates)

• Bare legs or, worse yet, bare feet shown off in sandals

• Fingernails so long folks wonder if you can shake hands without slashing their wrists

• Slit or wraparound skirts that fall open when you sit or walk

• *CLASSICS ARE ALMOST FOREVER* •

You can count on some styles to stay popular. For example, bikinis, jeans, T-shirts, tennis shoes, peasant blouses, and skirts are among the more enduring fashions. Poodle skirts, Nehru jackets, platform shoes, miniskirts, and pedal pushers are fads that have come and gone, as do all styles that go to fashion extremes.

Preppy is a term that will probably fade from use before the preppy fashions do. Basic pump heels and flats, shirtdresses, plaid wool kilts, wool blazers with brass buttons, polo shirts, pearls, and loafers are classics that can and will be worn for years.

If you stick to classics and stick to your diet, you can wear good clothing for years or at least until you change your life-style. I'm still wearing two good wool skirts ten years old, and my favorite pairs of jeans from college days.

• *SPECIAL-OCCASION DRESSING* •

The advice from wardrobe planning consultants is: never, never buy anything that is so "un-you" for a special occasion—party, job, interview—that you can never wear it comfortably again.

That does not mean you should never try a new look, but rather that you should consider your own personal style when buying any new clothing and accessories—unless, of course, you have money to spend on cluttering up your closets.

• *QUESTIONS* •

When you don't know what to wear—how dressed up or down you should be—ask! Ask the mother of the bride or groom what dress length is being worn at the wedding. Ask someone who's been with the company longer than you, preferably someone who's a step or two higher on the corporate ladder, what the appropriate dress is for company social functions. Call the hostess to find out if the party is casual or formal.

While you're at it, get the definition of "casual" if you are in an unfamiliar city or social stratum. We all know people who have gone to parties in jeans and tennies to find that "casual" meant not wearing a tie or cocktail dress. In Texas, there's a difference between dress jeans and regular, casual jeans. In New York or Boston, when someone says casual for dinner, I now know they don't mean my cowboy boots and slacks—which I almost wore once, but thank heavens I called the restaurant before leaving the house.

It's not dumb and embarrassing to have to ask about dress, but it sure makes you feel dumb and embarrassed when you are glaringly over or underdressed, *especially* when you are trying to make a good impression.

Sometimes you *can* recover. One of the great recoveries of all time occurred several years ago at a San Antonio patio party. In Texas, the dress for such an event is casual, meaning short-sleeved shirts for men and cotton dresses or slacks and flats or sandals for women; jeans are also worn.

One of the guests, a newcomer from the East Coast, misunderstood "patio" to be the same as a garden party and came to the party all gussied up in heels, mother-of-the-bride dress, and wide-brimmed hat. She was blessed with a great sense of humor, not to mention considerable poise, and each time she was introduced to someone as "Mary Jones, John's wife," she'd say, "No, that's wrong. I'm my twin sister, Sally Klutzheimer. She's the one who never does anything right."

And then, to top it off, she got her old sneakers from the trunk of her car, put them on with the garden-party outfit, and mingled with the other guests, starting conversations by talking about fashions and casual chic. Everyone remembered both of her names and she was the hit of the party.

Of course, a Sally Klutzheimer act wouldn't do if you were a new employee at a business social, but at a fun event it could even be more fun. Don't ever lose your sense of humor—it could help you through rough times.

• *DRESSING FOR SHOW AND TELL* •

If you have to speak before a group—your PTA, social club, business peers—ask yourself who will be there. What sort of people will they be—homemakers, buyers of products, good friends—and how will they be dressed? Where will I speak—in a church, a hotel dining room, a classroom/auditorium, the boardroom? What's the occasion? Is it serious or fun? Should *I* be serious or entertaining? I always try to dress about the same as the group I'm speaking to.

When I'm speaking at a convention in Hawaii, I dress casually. When it's a business group in Chicago, I wear a business suit. In Virginia, at a very old and prestigious club, I wore a hat—as did many women in the audience.

Do: wear a pretty color and/or something that draws attention to your face. Wear well-fitted, comfortable clothing appropriate to the occasion.

Don't: wear anything that requires constant adjusting or any jewelry that jingles and clangs against a microphone. Avoid stiff or itchy fabrics, too many layers of clothing that will make you feel too warm, and anything else that takes your—or your audience's—mind off what you want to say. (See the section in this chapter, "Looks That Have No Business at All.")

• DRESSING FOR A JOB INTERVIEW •

In addition to avoiding the "looks that have no business at all," wardrobe consultants advise against spending your first month's pay on an interview outfit, unless you can vary it enough to wear it to work repeatedly. The day before the interview, try on the whole outfit, including accessories, to make sure everything fits and looks right. Take your time—it's worth the effort. You might even want to walk around the room and sit down on a couple of different chair heights to test your mobility in the clothing and to practice shaking hands and saying hello. Above all, you want to make sure you feel comfortable in your outfit so that you can devote your energy and attention to making an impression on your prospective employer. You don't need any surprises, like buttons popping off a tight waistband while you're explaining why you'd be an asset to the company.

On the day of your interview get up extra early to give yourself plenty of time to dress. Tuck two extra pairs of pantyhose in your purse (three if you are run prone) just in case you get a run at the worst time.

• BUSINESS SOCIALS •

The general rule for business social dressing is that conservative companies dress conservatively even when at play, and trendy, flamboyant companies dress in flashier garb at work and play.

For women, a mid-calf-length dress in a darker color—black, navy, burgundy—that is not too sexy and revealing is safe at a black-tie event. Showing too much cleavage—or thigh—is a no-no if you or your husband are trying to climb the executive ladder.

Here's another tip: carrying a small handbag that you can gracefully tuck under your left arm when you shake hands with your right hand. Practice the handbag shuffle so that you won't look awkward when you meet Mr. or Ms. Bigwig.

Most of all, don't give up and stay home because you haven't a thing to wear. Better to be underdressed than to miss an opportunity to get to know the right people better.

• THE OLD SUPERSPEEDY SWITCHEROO GAME •

When you have a date after work, when you are traveling and just have time to pop in and out of your hotel room before going to dinner, when you've been out all day and come home to find that you and your spouse have surprise plans to go out for the evening, here's what to do.

Wrap a gold, glittery, or otherwise colorful belt around your dress or skirt or blouse.

Slip off your sensible shoes and slip on some sandals to perk up your feet. (Give them a quick wipe with a premoistened towelette, dab with a cotton ball saturated in astringent or alcohol, or a spray of cologne. They'll dry while you are freshening up your makeup.)

Change from your clunky, functional handbag to a small evening bag.

Top your everyday outfit with a velvet or silk blazer; put a glittery pin on its lapel. Or you can drape a shawl or a cape over your shoulders.

If you're wearing a shirtwaist dress or shirt-style blouse, undo an extra button for a less conservative look.

Change jewelry.

Put a pretty comb or barrette or other dressy ornament in your hair, which you can flip to one side or put up in the back for a fresher look.

If you have a little advance warning that you're going to have to play the old superspeedy switcheroo game, wear a silk dress to work that morning instead of a casual cotton; or a suit of soft, dark, dressy fabric instead of something sporty; or a collarless blouse or dressy camisole under your blouse so that you can just slip your blouse off. (This is my trick when I'm traveling.) If you are going out directly from the office, slip a camisole into your purse along with extrasheer stockings, a small evening bag, a change of jewelry, hair ornaments, and belt.

Remember, it's what shows above the table at the restaurant or while you are seated in the theater that counts—jewelry, camisole, hair/makeup repair, jacket, shawl, blouse. If that looks good, so will you.

If you keep an office emergency kit, you'll be able to repair almost any part of you that falls apart during the day. The kit should contain: needles, thread, safety pins, extra pantyhose, and colorless nail polish to stop runs in hose, nail clipper and file, spot remover, comb or hairbrush, clothes brush or used cellophane tape wrapped around your hand sticky side out to get rid of lint, tissues, spare lipstick or gloss, fold-up raincoat and/or hat.

• *DRESSING FOR TWO* •

If you are bored with ordinary maternity clothes and don't have the time or know-how to sew your own, there *are* things you can do.

Shop around for caftan/tent dresses in Indian or Mexican stores to find clothes that don't yawn "ho-hum."

Look for shirts and sweaters in the men's department and then donate them to the daddy when you are finished with them. Or if the man in your life shares, borrow some of his sweaters and shirts or elastic-waisted sweatpants. Look for men's jogging shorts in stretchy knits that will stretch your wardrobe as you stretch your midriff.

Check out thrift shops for maternity or tent clothing, and try to trade clothing or borrow from friends. I know of some neighborhoods where you can always tell who is pregnant—she's the one in the community maternity wear.

Slacks can be drawstring-waisted or you can stitch a stretch panel from the sewing notions department into the fly of your jeans or other pants for early pregnancy cover-ups.

It's important to buy sensible shoes for comfort and safety. Remember, you are walking for two, and, after a while, it becomes a challenge in the grace-and-poise department.

Use makeup to accent your eyes, and accessories to call attention to your face. Shoulder pads in your tops will create a little more balance to your total look.

This is the time to go pastel with some frills (but not too much) for an extrafeminine look. At the very least it will get you a seat on the bus!

Chapter 16

WARDROBE PLANNING: MAKING MORE OF LESS

lthough I've given beauty and wardrobe planning a great deal of thought and have read books by, and consulted with, experts, I'm still not sure whether a woman should find and stick with the makeup, hairstyle, and/or fashion look that suits her, making it her trademark, or whether it's better to keep changing, adapting new looks to your own special taste and style.

But I do know one thing: few of us can afford to have a whole new "self" each season. We all have favorite comfy clothing that we keep until (and maybe even beyond) its expiration date.

Katharine Hepburn is a good example of a woman who does not change her look: upswept hair, turtleneck sweaters topped with shirt/jackets, and straight-legged pants. Her trademark look is always fashionable. Other stars, Liz Taylor for example, change their image quicker than the camera clicks.

Basically, my wardrobe-planning philosophy is the same as the philosophy you will find throughout this book: what is best for you —that which makes you feel comfortable and suits you and your life-style—is best for you!

Most of us probably have both trademark looks and looks that we've adapted as they've become trendy. Both approaches need planning so that we can enjoy the most fashion for the least amount of money.

For most of us, learning to plan a wardrobe means going back to basics, then embellishing the basics with accessories. Like any other plan, before we can work it out, we need to assess the situation, set goals, and then have at it.

• *SIZING UP YOUR SITUATION* •

Whether you are entering the work world from college, where you wore jeans and sweats (as I did when I started working with my mother in 1974), or reentering the work world from the home, where you didn't need office clothes, or are just trying to look your best on a budget, the best way to start is with an inventory. See what you have that you can keep, then list what you need to supplement it. (See Chapter 14, "Closets: Behind Closed Doors," for getting-organized ideas.)

After you clean out your closets, make an inventory chart of your wardrobe, listing coats, jackets, sweaters, blouses, skirts, pants, dresses, and individual accessories (shoes, bags, belts, scarves).

On the chart mark the item and its color, description, and what it can be worn with. When you see all the items listed in one column and check the corresponding columns showing their colors, descriptions, and mates, you'll have a clear picture of what you have and what you need to buy so that you can get more mileage from your wardrobe.

You will also be able to tell whether you have been buying shotgun style—colors, textures, and fabrics that don't pull together when you need them to. You may realize, as I did, that you have eight black blouses but only one brown one to go with a beige suit. You may find that you can dress for any occasion in winter, but that your wardrobe limits you to beachcombing in the summer.

If you plan to go trendy, it's a good idea, before you actually start buying, to look at fashion magazines to see if what's new is really for you, or can be adapted to you.

Check out store displays and ads to learn how to accessorize new styles. Note handbag and shoe shapes. Study ways to wear jewelry and scarves with new clothing silhouettes.

Visit the expensive designer departments of stores, and then go to the budget departments to look for adaptations of designer looks —silhouettes, colors, and trimmings (bows, belts, and buttons) that have the new in look. Learn how to upgrade a less expensive outfit with good-quality belts or buttons, a splash of color from a scarf, or real or good-looking costume jewelry.

An expensive coat can make a big difference in your total look. Remember, some people will only see your coat, not what's under it, in cool to cold weather. When planning a pennywise put-together wardrobe, an all-season raincoat, preferably one with a zip-in lining that fits comfortably over suit jackets, will get you through the year in most climates.

What category of clothing do you need most—work, travel, dress-up, play? Shop accordingly.

Do you rarely go anyplace where you need to be dressy? You may be better off with one basic black dressy dress that can be dressed up or down with scarves, jewelry, a smashing jacket, and other accessories. Just about every woman needs one basic dress—the dress she wears when she doesn't know and can't find out what the occasion calls for. Black is the most practical, and the color of my basic wardrobe, but yours could be a different, most flattering, favorite color.

What colors do you really like? The reason I have eight black blouses and only one brown one is that I don't really like brown. I prefer black and red as the basic colors for my wardrobe.

The colors you buy most are likely to be the ones you like and wear most. Sometimes when I look into my closet, I marvel at how many black and red garments I have accumulated over the years. But I also have a bright blue silk dress that I love to wear. I bought it on sale in a weak moment and, when I unfurled it from its package at home, I felt as if I had lost track of all reason and sanity. It really stands out in my closet amidst the practical basic blacks, but even practical people need to do something offbeat once in a while, don't you think?

• PENNYWISE PUT-TOGETHERS •

My travel wardrobe and the basic working wardrobe suggested by most wardrobe-planning consultants are almost the same. The difference between a travel and basic working wardrobe is that you have more tops and bottoms and accessories at home than you would ever bother to take along on a trip.

A working wardrobe of a basic suit or blazer, two or three skirts, a couple of blouses, shirts, and sweaters, a dress or two that can be worn with the blazer or suit jacket, and a couple of basic accessories will, if they are in coordinating colors, combine for a variety of looks that multiply like the biblical loaves and fishes.

The key word here is *coordinating*. If your closet looks like a rainbow, chances are, when you try to mix and match, all you get is a mix instead of a match, definitely not a pennywise put-together.

Once you decide which color is your basic, it's easy to build on it. For example, my basic color is black (others include navy, burgundy, beige, brown), so my major wardrobe components, such as a suit or blazer and skirt, are black.

To expand upon a basic black suit or blazer and skirt, you can add blouses and scarves in white, cherry red, and blue in the summer, and light gray, beige, or burgundy blouses, sweaters, and scarves in the winter.

Textured and patterned skirts, pants, and dresses that expand on the basic color and mix well with it can then be added as you can afford them. Keeping with the "expansion" colors, add a textured or solid sweater-jacket, and keep expanding your pennywise put-together wardrobe, which will always be ready when you are, just like the airline commercial touts. This is especially true if you buy garments made of season-spanning fabrics.

• A COLOR-COORDINATED WONDER WARDROBE FOR WORKING WOMEN •

Using my basic black, here are the bare bones basics to cover your bare bones for work:

• *One coat:* your coat should be a color that coordinates with your wardrobe. I could wear black, white, or red with my basic black. Fur goes with all colors!

• *One suit:* my basic suit is black. Other basic colors include navy, burgundy, beige, or brown.

• *Blazer:* I would choose a black blazer that would mix and match with skirts, blouses, and my dress if I didn't have a black suit. My second blazer or jacket is gray.

• *Skirts:* colors, textures, and patterns of skirt fabrics should co-ordinate with the blazer, suit jacket, and tops. Three skirts will provide many different outfits. If you have a suit, count its skirt as one of the three you'll use when you start mixing and matching. I have gray, long black, and print skirts that go with my blazers, tops, and suit jacket.

• *A vest:* a red, black, or gray corduroy vest would go well with a black, gray, and white plaid or tweed skirt, and it could be topped with a black blazer.

• *Three sweaters:* sweater colors mix and match like blouses and scarves. (See below.)

• *Three to five good blouses:* among the blouse colors I can wear with my basic black suit (or black blazer and coordinated skirt) are white, red, and blue in the summer and light gray, red, or burgundy in the winter. Print blouses can be accented with solid-colored scarves and vice versa.

• *One dress:* my favorite traveling dress is a solid black that looks good with or without any color suit jacket. I also have black dress slacks to wear with or without my black jacket.

• *Two pairs of shoes:* black leather pumps and a second pair of shoes in neutral beige will go with just about any color combination you put together. I can accent my basic black with red shoes too.

• *One handbag:* if black is your basic, a good-quality black hand-bag will look smart every day.

• *Boots:* like shoes, a neutral color will give you the most mile-age. My black or gray boots go with my basic black wardrobe.

Here are wardrobe additions that you can add when you have accumulated enough money to cover checks you write for the clothes to cover you:

• *Unconstructed jacket:* I have a white-and-black jacket that goes with at least all of my skirts and three dresses.

• *Sweater-jacket:* a black-and-white, tweedy sweater-jacket tops a black skirt or black or white slacks. I wear a blouse for daytime and a camisole for evenings.

• *BEYOND BASICS: WARDROBE EXPANSION* •

As your finances allow, you can build on or, if you like, start another pennywise put-together unit with another basic color. A navy suit or navy blazer and skirt would be expanded with some of the same white, cherry red, green, gray, beige, or burgundy expansion items in your basic black unit. So, you see, a wardrobe can develop without your selling the family heirlooms to look good.

One fashion consultant estimates that a basic wardrobe of separates in year-round fabrics and colors, such as a wardrobe of two jackets, four skirts, five blouses, three sweaters, two vests, and two pairs of pants could be mixed and matched to form more than one hundred outfits, and that it would be almost four months before you went to work in a "rerun" outfit.

• *DOES IT WORK?* •

If you doubt that this working wardrobe really works, try to remember what a leading female politician was wearing that last time you saw her on TV. You don't recall? That's the point. People don't really remember what other people are wearing unless it's flashy or extremely unusual.

Believe me, if you switch sweaters and blouses, wear the dress with or without the blazer, you can create plenty of new looks.

Add to your basic wardrobe at sales. I always wait for sales, especially since I found out that most merchandise is marked up 100 percent! Sale prices are the best expansion for your wardrobe without damaging your checkbook.

If you are not the suit type, and have found your place in the workplace and don't feel as if you have to wear the dress-for-success uniform every day, you can still look tailored and businesslike if you shop around for softer fabrics and lines.

Try combining skirts with belted sweaters, or wear vests that coordinate with your blouses and skirts. Some sweater-jackets are as classic as suit jackets, but are stretchier and easier to wear for some women. Tweedy blazers or sweaters can coordinate with skirts and blouses for a business look.

Shirtwaist dresses are classics that go almost everywhere on almost anyone. (I avoid skirts that are too full because they aren't slimming.) If the fabrics are compatible, you can change the look of a shirtwaist dress by wearing a camisole or turtleneck sweater under it and leaving more buttons open down the front than you would when wearing only the dress. Jumpers have a finished look and may be more slimming to some women than the two-piece skirt-and-top look.

• *SPAN SEASONS TO STRETCH WARDROBES* •

In southern Texas, where I live, dark cottons have always been worn throughout the year because the climate is so warm. To meet today's demands across the United States, fashion designers have come up with clothing they call "season spanning" or "transitional," which can be worn throughout the year. The key to success for a year-round wardrobe is to coordinate the weights of fabrics. For example, you wouldn't wear a wool or velvet jacket with a gauzy cotton skirt unless the office in which you work is so cold that anything goes for your health's sake!

Do you remember when there was no air conditioning? We wore light fabrics in the summer or melted from the heat. Working or living in air-conditioned buildings means needing more than thin cotton gauze to survive. You can wear jackets and other wraps indoors in all seasons. Improved knits and cotton or wool jerseys are worn throughout the year. Dark cottons are worn year-round in cooler climates, too. Among the year-round colors are my favorites: red, navy, periwinkle blue, purple, and olive green.

Any neutrals, such as black, brown, beige, and putty, in fabrics ranging from cottons and linens to lightweight worsted woolens and wool crepe, gabardine, or silk, can be part of your wardrobe all through the year. Corduroy, Ultrasuede, and velour are also among year-round fabrics.

If you can't afford good natural fibers, choose good synthetics. Natural fibers breathe better than synthetics, and that's why they are better choices for year-round wear. Good choices for year-round wearing are such synthetic substitutes as polysilk, polyester, and rayon.

Blends of natural and synthetic fibers travel well and are a blessing to women who have little time to spare in the laundry room or driving to and from the dry cleaner. In the past few years, some of the travel problems with clothing made from natural fibers have been solved by designers who have made the wrinkled linen/cotton/ silk look not only acceptable, but definitely in.

Before you buy, remember to read care labels on clothing to determine how it is to be laundered or cleaned. You may prefer washables to dry cleanables because they're cheaper in the long run. I have a friend who says she ought to declare a certain silk dress she bought on sale a dependant on her income tax because she's spent so much money dry cleaning it.

· WARDROBE PLANNING ON A DAILY BASIS ·

After you have assembled your pennywise put-together wardrobe color-coordinated mixes and matches, you may find you can't get up in the morning and pick one from the more than one hundred combinations in your closet—at least not before morning coffee, and maybe not even then. It's like trying to diet at a Sunday brunch buffet in your town's fanciest hotel.

The trick is to do your mixing and matching the night before. Setting aside five minutes to put yourself together the night before is the best way to prevent mix-and-match mania—a trauma you suffer if you are still assembling the component parts when the carpool arrives and it's Irma Impatient's turn at the wheel—and the horn.

Another trick is to take some time every few weeks, or when the seasons change, to play with your clothing—to try out different combinations and arrangements of pins, scarves, and other accessories. The bonus: you'll get a fresh look that prevents you from dashing out and committing the sin of impulse buying. Those who are list makers, like me, make lists of new clothing combinations. Some people don't like lists, and that's okay too, as long as memory replaces the written list.

If you don't remember to or simply won't lay out your over and undergarments, shoes, and other accessories, plus anything you need to take with you the next day, here's an emergency put-together idea: just grab everything that is the same color and put it on—different textures for blouse, skirt, shoes, and any other accessories will usually blend together when they're the same color. You may not achieve a dramatic look, but it will probably be safe and acceptable—and will get Irma Impatient's palm off her beeping horn.

• *PENNYWISE PLAY WARDROBE* •

A play wardrobe can be assembled inexpensively by creative shopping. Often men's fleecy knit shorts, pants, and shirts are much cheaper than those you find in the women's department. They may not be in pastel pink and lavender, but, come on now, they *are* called sweats. Gray and navy aren't all that bad. You will find brighter colors in men's and boy's more expensive blend/knit jogging outfits and sweat suits.

The bonus, you'll soon see, is that buying male active sportswear usually gets you better quality for less money. Somehow, that seems unfair, doesn't it? It's just like free clothing alterations, which are almost always offered on men's clothing, but almost never on women's.

• *COLOR CONSULTATIONS* •

In most parts of the United States, women and men are using the services of professional color consultants who determine which colors and color "seasons" are best for their complexions. Some people have had satisfying results; others have been disappointed.

Some fashion writers who tested color consultants in their cities received conflicting color advice. For example, one consultant said a writer had rosy skin tones, and another said her skin was a peachy skin tone, each of course requiring different wardrobe colors.

Here's how to judge a color consultant's qualifications. Does he or she have proof of a one- to two-week, full-time training seminar with a recognized local or national color-consulting firm? Has the training included actual practice or just lectures? Also, does the color consultant have a background in related fields, such as art, fashion, cosmetology? Has he or she been in business for at least six months—with a firm or alone?

How much time will you have for consultation? Most experts say you should get, at the very least, one and a half hours. Naturally, you won't get that much individualized attention in a group session. Will follow-up service be included in the fee or will you have to pay extra for it? Some consultants arrange swap sessions so clients can trade clothing that no longer fits into their color-coordinated lives.

Generally, it's considered more effective if the consultant drapes you with fabric instead of choosing your colors from paint chips. Color selections *must* be made in natural sunlight or under daylight bulbs to be certain colors match your true skin tones.

You should be given a range of thirty to sixty color choices, plus suggestions on how to put them together and, preferably, additional advice on fashion and makeup.

Don't expect miracles. A consultant who promises them should be avoided, just as you would avoid a weight-loss program that guarantees a perfect figure in ten days or less. Finally, don't limit yourself to the color swatches you paid $50 to $300 or more for. Sometimes a shade that's a little off will work and will spare you chasing all over town to get a perfect match. Getting your colors charted is supposed to make your life rosy, not give you the blues. If you get carried away with trying to match everything perfectly, you might end up getting really carried away—to a rest home!

Chapter 17

ACCESSORIES: HINTS AND HOW-TOS

hen I travel, whether it's for two days or two weeks, my accessories help me create enough different looks out of my basic wardrobe so that I can hand carry all my luggage on the plane. A pin here, a scarf there, change of belt—all change the look of an outfit. What works for traveling works every day.

What makes a workable basic-accessory wardrobe? One good handbag (I've carried the same black bag for a year and a half), two pairs of shoes, three scarves, a watch, a bracelet, two pairs of earrings, two simple necklaces (pearls and gold go with everything), and two or three belts. If your belts match your shoes, you'll get a more finished look. Optional additions are a briefcase (if you use one), and for dress-up, evening shoes, a small, flat bag, and jewelry.

The main rule for accessories is "less is more." If I look in the mirror and wonder if I'm overdoing accessories on my outfit, then the answer is yes. It's the old "when in doubt, take it off" theory. It'll get worn another day. Too much clutter makes people look at your clothes instead of you.

· PENNYWISE PUT-TOGETHER ACCESSORIES WARDROBE ·

Belts

If your waist is a bit full, avoid wide belts. For a longer line, try wearing your belt a little lower than your natural waistline or wearing a thin belt at your hip line. You can even go one step farther—wear two thin belts, one on the hip and one a little higher.

For a belt from leftovers, try the hem fabric cut from a too-long skirt. It can be turned into a cummerbund or belt.

Boots

If you can, cuff the tops of soft boots or stuff your pants into boot tops for a knicker look. Be sure you have the right shape from *behind* for this look!

Briefcases

You can tuck your lunch, a small clutch bag, and your makeup kit into your briefcase—which by the way can also serve as an overnight bag in a pinch. I've seen some soft-sided briefcases that come with a small matching clutch bag that fits inside the briefcase pocket. You can remove the clutch and leave the briefcase in the office when you want to go out to lunch without taking your business with you.

Look for briefcases in handbag departments as well as in luggage departments; some are more feminine, others more functional. Hard-sided briefcases are good for keeping papers flat, but not so good for handling your lunch or a tape recorder.

Camisole

Make a camisole from an old sweater, T-shirt, or sweatshirt by cutting a straight line from underarm to underarm and stitching a fold wide enough to accommodate the elastic you'll insert in the channel. Thread elastic through the fold to gather the top and keep it up. Or, if the sweater or shirt bottom is tight enough, be lazy. Cut off the top and sleeves, turn the sweater or sweatshirt upside down so that the waistband is over your bust line, and tuck the rough cut edge into your jeans.

Catalog Accessories

If you aren't sure about accessorizing an outfit you've bought from a catalog, buy the accessories pictured with it in the catalog. They probably lured you into buying the outfit to begin with. Accessories can turn a plain-Jane dress into a gorgeous-gal outfit.

Coat-Dress Coat

Wear a coat-dress as a coat over a color-coordinated skirt and sweater.

Collar Up

To perk up your suit, pull your blouse collar out from under your suit jacket and then raise it and your jacket collar together for a stand-up, stand-out look. Add a scarf if you wish. Once, way before it was fashionable, I did this for a photo. The gentleman standing next to me took it upon himself to turn my collar down!

Earring Stick-ups

Use a leftover pierced earring to hold the rolled-up sleeves of a blouse if they won't stay put. Pierced earrings can hold a scarf in place, too, and serve as emergency buttons or tie clasps.

Funky Flea-Market Finds

Not everything at flea markets is for the house, and many household items found in the dusty bins can be converted into unique accessories.

Make an evening bag from any favorite fabric, and that includes antique napkins and hankies from flea-market sales. Your evening bag won't hold everything you keep in your everyday satchel, but it will hold keys, tissues, and pin money.

Make a belt from old silver- and copper-trimmed horse bridles.

Buy fancy belt buckles, then add your own fabric or leather

strips. If you're really feeling creative, braid the leather or fabric strips.

Sometimes drapery tieback cords can be turned into necklaces or belts. Often made from satin cord or velvet fabric, drapery tiebacks or servant bell cords can turn a plain basic dress or blouse into a knockout. Drapery departments in stores have silk cords that you can turn into belts or braid into your hair.

Web belts from old military uniforms can be nifty additions to slacks and jeans. If you don't hit the flea markets, you can buy new military items at army surplus stores.

Old table linens and dresser scarves can be turned into vests, and I have seen some great lacy tops made from old tablecloths.

Lingerie from the 1920s was often made of real silk, and today some people wear this lingerie at cocktail parties. Lacy bed jackets from the flapper era can double as blouses or vests.

Good men's shirts in wool, flannel, or cotton can make great baggy jackets for casual wear. Roll up sleeves if they are too long. Men's shirts also make good bathing suit cover-ups. You can often find good wool hunting shirts in army surplus stores or in sporting goods stores at the end of hunting season.

Buy an old knapsack at the flea market and use it to carry your finds, instead of dragging around bags. In fact, why not just buy a new knapsack for shopping? It no longer means you're a hippie, and it helps you distribute weight better on your back without weighing down arms. Also, a knapsack leaves your hands free to dig out more bargains.

Handbag Clutter

Use an old eyeglass case to hold the little things cluttering up the bottom of your purse—pens, pencils, comb, nail file, etc.

Lace It All Up

Dress up a plain outfit with lacy stockings, a lace hankie in a pocket, or a lacy camisole under a jacket.

Pin-up for Pins

For an unusual look, hang a pin on a choker necklace.

Place a pin in an out-of-the-ordinary place. I like to fasten one almost at my shoulder to draw the eye of the beholder upward.

Attach a pin to a length of grosgrain ribbon to make a choker. (Measure your neck first to determine the ribbon's length and include about six inches to tie a bow, less to tie a knot.)

I once met a woman who wore a family heirloom locket—a picture of her mother-in-law—on a ribbon choker. She joked that her mother-in-law was always at her throat.

Super Scarfery

Twist two scarves together and wear them as a belt or as a single scarf.

Wrap a print scarf around your waist, then over it buckle a belt that picks up on one of the scarf's colors.

Make an ascot from a long scarf by wrapping it twice around your neck, then flipping the ends over like an ascot; optional addition is a pin to the flap.

Tie a scarf in a bow, but instead of wearing it dead center in front, add a little flair by sliding the bow off toward your shoulder —even *on* the shoulder, if you feel like it.

Use a scarf as a cummerbund. Unless you're a Scarlett O'Hara, a fifty-four-inch length is best for belting, and a smaller forty-five-inch scarf will work better at your neck.

Small square scarves can flash color from a jacket pocket or be folded on the bias and tied behind your neck to look like an ascot; larger scarves tied this way can be worn outside of a blouse or sweater.

Tie a scarf on the outside of your coat to brighten it up; for real pizzazz, add a color matching your hat.

Knot an oblong scarf with a Windsor or men's tie knot, putting the knot at any level—high at the throat or low at the bust line.

Fold a square scarf on the bias and tie sailor or cowboy style.

Turn a square scarf into a jabot, and wear it inside or outside a blouse or dress collar by folding the square into an oblong shape, and then flipping one end over the other at your throat. Add a pin or tie tack if you like.

Tie a small scarf to your handbag strap for a flash of color.

Stockings

I like my stockings to be one shade lighter than my shoes. Most fashion experts agree that stockings that coordinate with your skirt will pull your look together. If your skirt is too short, matching hose will make it seem the right length. I like wearing colored, opaque, or textured hose with heavy-textured clothing such as tweeds or nubby wools.

Socks

Stuff your key, change, and hankie into the cuff of your sock if you don't want to carry a handbag while you're on a walk. If you are on a long hike and are toting all sorts of creature comforts, such as lip balm and a piece of hard candy, wear two pairs of socks and stash your stuff between the cuffs.

Cardigan Sweaters

A full-length cardigan sweater or one that falls below the hips can make an outfit look casually chic. You can even use a long sweater for a beach cover-up.

Swinging Sweaters

Toss a sweater over your shoulders and tie the arms at front and center for a color accent on the upper part of your body.

Belt your pullover when you wear it over pants or skirt.

Belt your cardigan after you have buttoned the last few buttons on the bottom to create a jacket look over a blouse or turtleneck.

• NEAT IDEAS AND EMERGENCY FIXES •

Lost Belts

Here's where a stitch in time really saves nine. Before you lose the matching belt to a dress, coat, robe, or suit, get out your needle and thread and either tack the belt to the belt loops or tack it to the center back of the garment.

Black and White

Shiny black patent handbag or shoes will add sparkle to a dull outfit. Try accenting last year's blouse with a black ribbon or sheer fabric bow or tie. Add a white collar to a collarless blouse, sweater, or dress. A black-and-white print or striped scarf can top a black dress.

Bras

Flesh-colored bras don't show through sheer blouses the way white ones do. Underwires that poke out of underwire bras can be quickly covered with a piece of moleskin or tape.

Errant Earring Backs

I once lost an earring back on my way to do a live TV show. There was no time to dash into a dime store to buy a cheap pair of earrings so that I could use its stud back, so I found a tiny piece of cork and stuck it in the back of my earring. Believe it or not, that piece of cork stayed in place all day long!

For another emergency earring back, cut the eraser off of a pencil.

Peek-a-Boo-Blouse

If the buttons on your blouse front are positioned so you have a slight gap over the bust line when you move your arms, try some of the following suggestions.

Tie a scarf in a sailor knot, so that the knot is positioned right over the gap.

Knot a long necklace so the knot hides your peek-a-boo.

Put a pin at the gap.

Pull it all together from the underside of your blouse with a safety pin, and use a scarf or necklace to cover the dimple made by the pin.

If the buttons on a blouse are not positioned properly (if there isn't a button right at the bust line), don't buy the blouse.

Summer Dress

You can turn a long, elastic-waisted cotton skirt into a strapless summer dress by pulling the waist above your bust line and adding a colorful belt. You also can get a full-slip effect from a half-slip by pulling the half-slip waist up over your bust line when you need a quick cover-up under a sheer blouse.

Softening Handbags

If you've stored a plastic handbag in a scrunched position, you can puff it back into shape by blowing hot air from a hair dryer into it. Then, when the plastic softens, shape it up and back to its original form.

Keeping Your Hem Dry

There are at least two ways to keep the hem of a long dress out of rain or snowy wetness. Either cut two holes in an extralarge garbage bag, step inside, pull up the bag, and secure it to your waist with a belt; or tie a cord around your waist and pull up your gown over it to form a short blouson. You probably wouldn't want to walk into a fancy country club in a garbage bag, but if you were going to a wedding and had to arrive clothed, you wouldn't think twice about protecting your dress, would you?

Cold Night, Warm Nightie

On a cold night, toss your night clothes into the dryer for a few minutes before you put them on for a comfy feeling treat.

Padding on Your Account

In an advice column, I once read that what nature has forgotten, you can always stuff with cotton. If nature has forgotten to give you shoulders, or you want to change the line of a blouse or dress, you can fill in sloping shoulders with shoulder pads. (Fooled you! Bet you thought I was going to suggest bra stuffing.)

Pants Lint

If your pants legs gather lint and pet hair when you walk across your rug, spray them with antistatic spray or rub them with fabric softener sheets *before* you trek out of your bedroom. Use the same technique when you have a clinging skirt. To prevent static, add one tablespoon of white vinegar to the final rinse water when you wash static-prone garments.

Something Up Your Sleeve

If your blouse sleeves are too long, cuff them. If jacket sleeves are too long, do the same, then fold the cuff of your long-sleeved blouse back up over the sleeve for a show of inner color. Or roll the blouse and jacket edges and give them a push up for a casual look. Be sure it looks right and not like a "make-do."

By the way, the correct sleeve length is just long enough to cover the top of your wristbone. The shirt sleeve should peek out an extra quarter of an inch.

Stuck with Stockings

If you can't pull up pantyhose that are too short, wet your hands with water and rub the legs upward. They should roll right up. Next time, stretch them lengthwise before putting them on.

Stocking Spatters

If your stockings get spattered in the rain, wipe off those splotches with wet paper towels. Spatters tend to be so irregular, you can't get away with pretending that they're the texture of your textured hose, can you?

Stocking Preservation

If you are one of those folks whose toes poke through hose before you put your shoes on, try pulling the toe of your hose to stretch it away from your big toe; the extra room will help prevent piercing. One of my readers has suggested putting a one-inch piece of half-inch-wide first-aid tape on each big toe. Place the tape about a quarter-inch down from the toenail edge; smooth it over the nail, the nail edge, and then down the back of your toe.

Shoes

Leather shoes will last longer if you keep the leather preserved with shoe cream or polish. Consider new lifts on the heels of new shoes as a preventive measure before they wear down to the main part of the heel. There's no friend as comfortable as an old shoe, so help your friend have a longer life. Check with your shoe repair service;

synthetic lifts that last much longer than leather can even be put on your *new* shoes.

Waistband Emergency Expansion

If you put on a skirt or pants and then find that your waistline has expanded, let a short length of very narrow elastic come to your rescue. Tie it into a loop, using a knot that won't slip. Slip-knot one end to the buttonhole and loop the other end around the button. Cover your sins with an overblouse and resolve to start that diet and begin your exercise regimen.

• SPOT AND STAIN REMOVAL •

If spot remover, detergent, and/or bleach won't take a spot out of washable fabrics, hot sun and lemon juice will. And if you can't get the spot out at all, and your dry cleaner can't either, you can cover it up with an appliqué or pin.

Stains get set in the laundry so often that it's a good idea to establish a method of identifying spotted garments, such as a knot in the sleeve or attaching a clothespin or safety pin before tossing the garment in the hamper. Some of my friends who have large families don't like the knot in the sleeve idea because they say spot-prone children would end up with totally knotted up clothing that would take hours to untangle for washing.

If you can, get your family to spot-clean stains before they toss clothing into the hamper. The mother of a large family told me that this is not practical; she is still working on getting her teenagers to toss their clothing into the hamper!

There are no guarantees when it comes to spot or stain removal because the type of stain, fabric, and the amount of time the stain has to set all vary so much that no one method is guaranteed to work. But a garment that has an ugly stain on it is not wearable anyway, so what can you lose? You like to feel as if you have tried, so on with it. I think any stain on a very expensive garment is best treated by a professional cleaner who has all sorts of chemicals and time-learned techniques at its disposal.

Before you try any method of spot or stain removal, read the care label on the garment so you'll know how to treat the fabric. See section on care labels in Chapter 17, "Let's Go Shopping."

The basic rule for stain removal is: always keep another cloth under the stain being worked on to absorb the "remover" and the "removee" mess. The cloth should be white so that no color will run onto the garment to complicate the situation. Always blot with clean white cloth; don't rub.

Here are some techniques that prevent your cure (removal) from being worse than the complaint (stain):

Test any stain-removing chemical on an inconspicuous part of the garment.

Take nonwashable garments to the dry cleaner immediately and be sure to tell the clerk what the stain is.

Apply cleaning fluids to insides of fabrics. Some essential stain-removal aids are a good general cleaning fluid, some type of bleach and hydrogen peroxide for fabrics that can be bleached, ammonia, turpentine, prewash, presoak products. If a garment can be bleached, dishwasher detergent paste works really well. (Make the paste by wetting the fabric and sprinkling on the detergent; scrub with an old toothbrush; wash in hottest water possible, depending on the type of fabric.)

Alcoholic Drinks

Rinse as soon as possible—or sooner—with a white vinegar and cool water solution; launder according to fabric requirements.

Antiperspirant

Blot the spot with a paper towel moistened with a vinegar or baking soda solution; you may need to soak the garment for best results. Wash it in hottest water safe for the fabric, and add extra bleach.

Ball Point Pen Ink

Alcohol removes ball point pen ink on washable fabrics most of the time. You can also spray the ink stain with hair spray (alcohol is among its ingredients), apply nail polish remover (if it is safe for the fabric), or use prewash products, all of which are effective on some inks. Follow treatment with appropriate laundering method.

Blood Stains

Several techniques work; try the one best suited to the fabric.

Flush with cold water; apply liquid detergent.

Dampen and sprinkle with unflavored meat tenderizer and let sit. Or, if fabric can be bleached, pour on hydrogen peroxide and let the peroxide bubble away; rinse with cool water.

Soak in cool water with a sprinkle of table salt added; wash with gentle soap in warm water.

Soak in cool water about an hour at least; rub with bar soap and launder.

Persistent stains may come out with soaking in a cold water solution consisting of two tablespoons ammonia to one gallon water; followed by washing and bleaching, if the garment can be bleached.

Candle Wax or Crayon

This works with washable fabrics: chip off as much of the hardened wax as possible with your fingernail, a dull knife, or credit card. Then place paper towels on either side of the waxed area, and iron on a low to medium setting, depending on the fabric. If any stain remains, apply liquid detergent and water or dry-cleaning solvent; rinse and wash as usual.

Candy (Not Chocolate)

Rub a little detergent on the stain; rinse with cold water. For stubborn red stains, soak item in strong laundry detergent and a little bleach (if fabric can be bleached); or treat with prewash spray.

Catsup

Blot up as much as possible. Rinse or soak in cold water. Spray with prewash product. Sometimes liquid detergent will remove catsup.

Chewing Gum or Adhesive Tape

Scrape off excess with dull knife (this is easier if you put the garment into the freezer or rub an ice cube over the gum to make it more brittle); remove remainder with a cleaning fluid that's appropriate to fabric. Prewash spray squirted on the back of a stain on washable fabric after the solid part is removed usually will work.

Chocolate

Apply prewash spray, ammonia, or sometimes hydrogen peroxide (if it's safe for fabric); work solution into fabric; let it set; rinse in cold water; wash.

Coffee or Tea

Rinse in cold water; bleach if fabric can be bleached or use nonchlorine powdered bleach on stain. After spot treating, wash in the hottest water safe for fabric. This is one of the exceptions to the rule of using cold water on all spots to avoid setting the stain.

Cosmetics

Wet stain and rub with bar soap. If the stain remains, work undiluted liquid detergent into the spot and launder as usual.

Fruit

As soon as you can, flood stain with cold water and treat with prewash spray. If stain has dried, soak garment in cool water; work detergent into the stain and rinse. Use color-safe bleach in laundry.

Fruit Juices, Cocktails, Other Beverages

Do not use soap. Remove stain with liquid detergent or hydrogen peroxide bleach. Some fruit stains can be removed with a solution of ammonia and water, followed by laundering according to fabric.

Grass

There are several methods for taking out grass stains:

If material is bleach-safe, use bleach according to directions. If it's not, use nonchlorine bleach or hydrogen peroxide; soak; launder as usual.

After applying ammonia and cold water to the stain, let it soak overnight in presoak detergent.

Grease

Here are three ways to remove grease:

Treat with commercial degreaser product.

With a white cloth placed under the stain, apply cleaning fluid appropriate to the fabric to the reverse side of fabric; rub with bar soap or liquid detergent; wash in hot water.

Shampoo will remove some types of grease. A good tip for travelers: sponge stain out with shampoo, rinse and then dry with hair dryer, and you're ready to tour.

Lipstick

Treat with prewash product; rub spot with clean paper towel; repeat procedure until lipstick is removed. Then rub dampened stain with bar soap and wash. Rubbing alcohol works, too.

Mildew

The best mildew killers I know are lemon juice and salt, or white vinegar and salt. Place the treated clothing in the sun; after the sun has done its job, wash as usual. Always wash mildewed items separately to prevent it from spreading to other items. Did you know that lemon juice will sometimes remove a stain that appears to have set if used with the sunlight method?

Regular chlorine bleach works on certain fabrics; be sure to read the labels on fabrics and bleach *before* using.

Milk or Cream

Soak in warm water with presoak product.

Mustard

Apply peroxide or white vinegar. *Do not* use ammonia. Wash as usual.

Paint or Varnish

For best results, get to the stain before it dries. Place white cloth under stain; blot wrong side of fabric with turpentine, paint thinner, or other solvent compatible with the paint and fabric. Then soak garment in warm water and wash as usual, using extra detergent. Don't use turpentine on acetate fabric.

Perspiration

Using extra detergent, wash in hottest water safe for fabric. If the garment can be bleached, use bleach. Deodorant and perspiration stains on underarms should also be treated this way. If the garment has a lot of stain buildup, there may be no hope of getting it out.

Rust

Rub with lemon juice; let it dry in the sun; repeat if necessary; launder.

Urine

Soak stain in presoak product with a little bleach. Wash as usual. Sponging with diluted white vinegar or perborate bleach may restore the original color. *Caution:* do not use ammonia on diapers. Instead, use a borax solution; it prevents odors as it whitens and softens.

Vomit

Soak in cool water solution of one cup salt to one gallon water; rinse and wash. If the stain doesn't come out, you may also have to dab with white vinegar before you rinse and wash.

Wine

I pour club soda on wine stains, then rinse in cool water. If the material can be bleached, follow instructions. If the fabric can't be bleached, dishwasher detergent paste makes a great stain remover for wine or any other stain.

Yellowing of Bleachable Fabrics

Make a solution of one-half cup chlorine bleach and one tablespoon white vinegar to one gallon of warm water; soak at least an hour; repeat treatment if necessary; wash and dry in sunlight. Be super gentle with antique or vintage clothing that has yellowed or is stained.

· SHOES ·

Isn't it awful when your feet hurt? I can't think of anything that puts those frown lines on your face faster than poorly fitted shoes and tired, aching feet.

Fitting Shoes

Podiatrists tell us that as many as 92 percent of all people have some sort of foot problem. About 75 percent of those problems are corns and calluses caused by small spurs (bony calcium growths) on the bone. And what causes these spurs? Some you can blame on your ancestors; others are caused by the bone's reaction to a body chemistry that's out of balance, or the bone's reaction to pressure. And where does pressure come from? Badly fitted shoes.

Surgery will correct foot problems, but if you don't correct the reason for the problem, it will return. Crunched toes get corns. Pressure on your big toe bone can cause bunions.

Did you know that a bunion is not something that grows on your foot? A bunion is really a joint that has buckled from pressure, such as when you have a short first metatarsal bone (short big-toe bone), which buckles the joint where the toe bone connects to the foot bone. You need shoes that take the pressure off the joint and put it on the outer edge of your foot, where it belongs. And that means properly fitting shoes.

If your shoe fits properly, from the heel to the ball of your foot, your toes will take care of themselves, and your weight will be properly balanced on your shoe. Width, too, is important.

The arch of the shoe should support your arch. Those little foam pads you see in the arches of some shoes are not arch supports. They are really more for show than for function.

As your feet get older, arches weaken, and you may notice that your foot may grow as much as a half size, though it will be narrower due to your foot stretching forward. Shoe sizes also get larger if *you* get larger by gaining weight; in fact, many people find they need narrower shoes after they lose weight. I find that my cowboy boots get tight when I put on about seven pounds. Actual foot growth stops at about age eighteen in women and about nineteen in men.

Podiatrists seldom have anything good to say about high-heeled shoes, but we wear them anyway. Fortunately, in the past few years, fashionable shoes with lower heels have become more popular.

Have you ever wondered why high heels make feet feel tired and achy? Normally, 65 percent of our weight is on our heels and 35 percent is on the forefoot. When heels go up, our weight is shifted forward to the balls of our feet, which simply were not designed to hold all that weight. The changes you make in your posture to maintain balance on high heels, podiatrists say, also strain your back. Lower-back pain and all sorts of abdominal complaints result. Eventually, your body adapts to the switch, but your feet still suffer. To be sensible, alternate heel heights. Constant wearing of high heels will shorten your calf muscles; and negative-heel shoes, so popular a few years back, actually cause torn calf muscles—especially in folks who inherited shorter calf muscles.

Heel heights of one and a quarter to two inches are usually comfortable for daily wear. If you just must wear those lizard spiked heels, save them for sit-down dinners.

Adjusting Fit

Absolutely nothing can be done to shoes that are too short, but some shoes can be stretched wider, and pads can be slipped into shoes that are too wide.

Most people's feet are not exactly the same length and width, so buy to fit the foot that feels most comfortable, and adjust the not-so comfy shoe. There is only one-twenty-fourth of an inch difference between an A and AA width. If neither is comfortable, *don't buy!* A shoe is no bargain at any price if it doesn't fit correctly.

Also, remember that different styles may mean different sizes: you may need to buy a larger size in pumps than you do in sandals.

Quality

Quality shoes are made from lasts (the plastic forms they're made on) that correspond exactly to each size and width. Cheaper shoes may be made in 7-narrow, 7-medium (or whatever) instead of 7-A, 7-AA, 7-AAA, and so on to 7-D. And like better and hand-tailored clothing, the more hand stitching, the better the fit.

Materials

Real leather uppers will conform and mold themselves to the shape of your feet better than man-made materials. Leather linings allow your feet to "breathe" more than man-made materials. Many people also prefer leather soles for comfort, and others prefer a spongy sole, especially if they're on their feet for long periods of time.

General Care Hints for Shoes

If you find a style you like in a color you like to wear almost daily, you can buy two pair and alternate them. Ideally, you should change shoes once or twice daily, because the acid in foot perspiration tends to deteriorate leather.

Shoes need to air between wearings; don't store them in plastic boxes or bags.

Use silicone spray to make your shoes water-repellent before they get wet.

Shoe repair shops can "take the slippery" off the soles of new shoes with a sanding machine. But you can sand the soles yourself with an emery board, fine sandpaper, or just wear the shoes outdoors and wipe your feet on the cement sidewalk—anything to prevent skidding on the first carpet you walk on.

Shiny spots on suede shoes can be roughened up with an emery board or piece of fine sandpaper. But rub lightly.

One of my readers solved the problem of squeaky shoes by putting two thumbtacks on the bottom of each shoe, under the arches on each side of a metal arch support.

Stretch tight shoes with homemade shoe trees made from jam or jelly jars—stuff them into the shoes to stretch them while they rest in the closet.

Polishing Shoes

Polish your shoes to keep leather soft and new-looking. And remember there is no "MEN ONLY" sign at shoe-shine stands; women can get a professional shine, too. Shoe repair shops offer a "finishing" service that can really renew a favorite pair of old shoes (or a handbag).

For a really spiffy shine, you can buff shoes with a floor polisher. Just turn the waxer on its side on a chair, apply shoe wax, and buff away!

For a quick shine, spray on furniture polish. Rub it in with your fingers and wipe off the excess with a towel. The polish helps prevent black marks on white shoes, too.

Use a clean pencil eraser to remove scuff marks on patent leather shoes.

Did you ever notice that wax polishers don't cover scuffs very well, and most liquids don't leave a nice shine? Try applying liquid polish first; let dry; then apply wax polish and buff. Old shoes look nice as new.

You can touch up the black edged soles (or heels) of shoes with permanent black marker. Be careful not to blacken the shoe leather itself, though.

Shoelaces

To figure out the length of the shoelace you need for replacement, count the number of holes in the shoe (on one side only) and multiply it by six. For example, if one side of the shoe has five holes, you'll need to buy thirty-inch laces.

When washing laces, such as those from tennis shoes, either remove them from the shoes and sprinkle with detergent and scrub with a toothbrush, or tie the laces through a skirt buttonhole and run them through the washer.

You can also clean laces by soaking them in a small jar filled with bleach and soap and water while the shoes are being washed in the machine.

Athletic Shoes

Consider all the ways you're going to use them—aerobic dancing, jogging, tennis—before you make your decision. The tops, support, and soles are all designed for specific purposes.

For example, runners tend to pronate (roll their ankles inward); a shoe that has extra support under the arch will help prevent pronation. Hiking boots lace up to the ankle to give it support and will have cleated (rubber these days, not metal) soles to provide more traction. Tennis shoes will have a smoother sole to accommodate asphalt. Some shoes will have information listed on box-tops, such as "not recommended for lateral motion," which means they are not suited for the racquetball courts. Find a shoe salesperson who knows something about athletic shoes and read the boxes the way you read food labels to get the shoe best suited for your needs.

To keep those tennies clean and new-looking, spray them with a soil repellent or spray starch when they are new, or after you have washed them. It will help keep dirt from getting ground in and they will be easier to clean.

For extraclean inner soles, scrub with detergent and a brush before tossing the shoes into the washer.

Dry sneakers by hanging them on the line by their tongues. (Sounds mean, doesn't it?) Or take a drapery hook; hook it through the top eyelet of the shoe, and then over the clothesline. Also, you can place your shoes in front of the fridge to let the warm air from the motor dry them.

Save your old, beat-up tennies for "river shoes"—the shoes you need when you are camping or picnicking in or around rivers and other messy places.

Mend sneakers by sewing those separated soles to the tops with fishing line for a few more wearings.

To keep your toe from wearing through sneakers, try putting a piece of adhesive tape inside the shoe, where your little toe or top of big toe rubs the side and toes will have to wait a little longer before they sneak out of your sneakers.

Boots

Rolled-up newspaper stuffed into your boots will keep the shank in shape while your boots aren't being worn.

Can't zip up your high boots? Hook the top of a wire clothes hanger into the zipper eye and pull.

Unlined rubber boots will slip on more easily if you spray the insides lightly with spray-on furniture polish. Of course, if the boots are too small, nothing will help.

Shoes to Look Good

Most fashion folks agree that leather, whether it's calf, lizard, or snakeskin, is the best look for most occasions.

Classic pumps supposedly are the most flattering to your legs. And pumps aren't just plain pumps anymore. New designs offer heel shapes and sizes and a variety of colors and styles that are equally appropriate at the office and a party.

In warm weather, sling-back pumps and open toes are fine for the workplace; in general it's wise to avoid strappy shoes that look too little girlish or partyish.

• *JEWELRY* •

Jewelry is the accessory that literally makes you sparkle. And although any accessory you wear is a matter of taste, working outside of the home often means not sparkling *too* much.

Earrings

Dangly chandelier-style earrings that seem glamorous at night are not really appropriate office wear, plus they'll probably get caught in the telephone cord.

Of course, you don't have to limit yourself to wearing the studs you got when you had your ears pierced. Earrings about the size of a nickel are usually acceptable even in the most conservative place of business.

When you're packing for travel, stick your pierced earrings into an index card or other card so you don't lose them.

Necklaces

You don't have to stick to the standard pearls or gold chains for business wear; other beads, such as garnets, lapis, and onyx, can add to your look. If you buy long strands, these can be worn as double-strand necklaces or knotted at one end for different looks. Twisting a pearl necklace and an equal-length strand of beads creates yet another look.

Once you've accumulated a collection of necklaces, do they crawl around in your jewelry box and get totally tangled up with each other so that getting them undone is more than you can deal with? One of my readers stuck several adhesive-backed plastic hooks on her dresser mirror, and now her necklaces stay right where she puts them—on the hooks, untangled and in view.

Necklaces can also be hung on corks nailed to the wall in or out of your closet.

To avoid tangles when you're traveling, wrap your chains around a hair roller and secure with a bobby pin. But don't pack your jewelry in your checked luggage; you may never see it again!

Bracelets

Clusters of bangles and chains can be just too distracting in an office when they clatter against desk tops and each other or, worse yet, get tangled in your earrings or necklace as you gesture to make your point in a meeting. I've learned not to wear dangling jewelry when, for example, I'm on radio shows. You wouldn't believe how much racket a few bracelets can make against a microphone! I suggest opting for a single band or bracelet.

Here's an idea for folks who have trouble putting—and keeping —a bracelet or watch with a clasp-type hook on. Those things just seem to slip off your wrist with a mind of their own, don't they? If you tape one end of the bracelet to your wrist, slowly bring up the other end, and then snap it in place, you'll have that bracelet or watch on with no fuss at all.

Pins

Lots of people have so much trouble deciding where to put a brooch or pin that they end up putting it back into the drawer. Try positioning your pins in different places when you have some play time instead of when you're rushing to get dressed for work or play.

As I've mentioned, I like to change the focus point of a suit or blouse by placing a pin high up on my shoulder—almost at the shoulder seam. This draws attention to my face, rather than my lapel.

General Jewelry Hints

If you have an allergic reaction to jewelry, such as a rash under a ring, or if the metal reacts with your skin and tarnishes, try several thin coats of clear fingernail polish painted around the inside of the band of a ring or bracelet and on the back of an earring.

Adding charms to a bracelet or a dangle to an earring? Put a drop or two of glue on the small ring opening and you won't need to solder it.

If you drop a tiny screw or a small stone from a piece of jewelry, fasten a piece of organdy or nylon stocking over the end of your vacuum hose with a heavy rubber band; run the vacuum over the area, making sure the hose is always covered.

Real Jewelry

If you like real jewelry—pearls and/or gold—but have a limited budget, why not save up and treat yourself to the real thing, then wear it with everything as your personal trademark? The alternative is to inherit real jewelry, but not all of us have wealthy ancestors.

My trademarks are my pearl rings and a gold leaf pin, all of which were my mother's, and which I wear 95 percent of the time. The pin has become my good luck charm. Once when I was zooming through an airport, I reached over to my left shoulder where I usually pin it to make sure I hadn't flipped it off with my shoulder bag, and mother's gold leaf wasn't there. I panicked! But then I looked over and saw that I had switched it that day to my right shoulder!

Costume Jewelry

It's here to stay, and I say as long as it goes with what you're wearing, go ahead and enjoy it. Colored plastic costume jewelry that's well made can perk up and accent your summer wardrobe. Polished wood costume jewelry goes nicely with hot- or cold-weather looks. Costume jewelry is fun, and it doesn't cost you a month's rent.

Jewelry Boxes

How many times have you looked into your jewelry box and wondered when you're going to get around to dusting it out? Well, here's an easy way: just cover the wand of your vacuum cleaner with nylon net or a stocking and then vacuum the box out—without having to dump out all your jewelry.

Making Your Own Jewelry

For a funky necklace-and-earring set, try stringing about eighteen one-and-a-half-inch colored square or round (or combination) wooden beads on a satin cord, knotting between each bead; then for matching earrings, thread some of the cord through a bead, knotting it at each end to cover the bead hole and glue the bead to an earring back. You'll find colored wooden beads in craft stores. This could also be made in wood tones with a brown or wood-tone cord.

Raid your local fishing tackle shop for costume jewelry. (You heard me right!) Get a box of fishing swivels, and string them together with satin cord, knotting the cord in between each swivel. You can make single or multitiered necklaces, and if you hook swivels onto earring wires for pierced ears, you'll have matching earrings.

You can use your imagination to create jewelry by gluing buttons, bows, beads, lace, shells, or anything else on earring backs or pins for special effects, and the cost is special, too. (I mean low!) Imagination is a great money saver.

Really Real versus Really Fake

A reputable store will appraise any jewelry it sells to you at the time of sale at no charge, but most will charge a small fee to give you any appraisals after that. Few stores will give free appraisals or any appraisals on jewelry that they haven't sold to you. In general, it's probably a better idea to get an independent appraiser, so that you'll get an unbiased view of the jewelry's value.

Look for an appraiser who has graduated from or has at least attended a reputable gem school, such as the Gemological Institute of America. Always save sales slips and appraisal notes for your insurance company in case you need to make a claim.

Jewel-Speak

Carat or Karat? Carat is the weight of a stone—diamond, ruby, sapphire, and so forth. It's usually abbreviated ct. with a number before it, such as .25 ct. or 1 ct. A carat has 100 points, so 25 points equals .25 carat. Five carats equal one gram in metric weights, and

142 grams equal one ounce—although you aren't likely to have contact with diamonds by the ounce unless you are a jeweler.

Karat is the term used to measure gold parts to alloy, i.e., the purity of gold. The more gold in jewelry, the softer the metal. Pure gold is 24-karat; 12-karat is half gold and half base metal. The lowest quality of gold that can be sold in this country is 10-karat. Most American jewelry is 14-karat or 14K gold, which means a piece is made from 14 parts gold to 10 parts of alloy.

If you shop for foreign-made gold pieces, you'll find that most European gold is 18K, and most Mexican gold is 10K. The karat value will be marked on quality gold jewelry, just as "sterling silver" is marked on silver pieces. Quality jewelry, if you can afford it, is a better buy.

"Solid gold" means that the piece is not hollow; the term does not refer to the karat of the gold.

"Gold-filled" (base metal rolled in a layer of gold) and "gold-plated" (base metal electronically plated with gold) jewelry, if rubbed hard enough, will show the base metal from which the piece was made. The layer of gold fused to electroplated gold is at least seven millionths of an inch thick. In this country the karat will be 10K or better.

Precious stones include agate, emeralds, garnets, jade, onyx, rubies, and sapphires.

Semi-precious stones include aquamarines, amethysts, tourmalines, and other stones less rare, and therefore less valuable, than precious stones.

Diamonds are the result of the wonderful thing nature did with carbon instead of turning it into coal! Size, cut, flaws, and color determine the value, and you need to trust your jeweler because many of the extraordinary new fake diamonds are so good. At one time a diamond's authenticity was determined by dropping it in a container of oil and seeing how quickly it sank, but the newer fakes react to this test just like real diamonds, so it is no longer valid.

Zircon, spinel, strontium titanate, cubic zirconia—all are names for fake diamonds. Some are colored to be fake precious or semiprecious stones. You will find cubic zirconia set in 14K gold quality mountings that pass for real; most of the cost is for the gold, which makes the stone look even more real. In fact, many people today are choosing the fakes—they're easier to care for and less bother when it comes to traveling, storage, etc.

If a grain of sand or other irritant finds its way into an oyster shell, the oyster automatically covers it to prevent irritation, and after a few years of this—*voilà!*—you have a pearl. If the irritant is one grain of sand or another particle and it happens accidentally, you have a "natural" pearl, very hard to find these days.

Cultured pearls account for most of the real pearls sold today, and the process is the same as for natural pearls, except that it's not mother nature who inserts the mother-of-pearl bead into the oyster's tissue—it's man. Two types of cultured pearls are fresh-water Mobe, which are usually round or oval-shaped, and the rare saltwater Keshi, which come in irregular shapes and colors.

Simulated pearls—beads of glass, plastic, or other materials coated with various substances, such as ground fish scales—are totally man-made. The finest of the simulated pearls are the Spanish-made Majorca pearls, which are dipped fourteen times for the best "pearly luster." The cheaper the simulated pearls, the fewer their layers of "pearl essence."

The luster of natural and cultured pearls seems to come from inside the pearl. You can tell the difference between cultured and simulated pearls by the shape; simulated pearls will all have the same shape. Also, if you rub cultured pearls against your tooth, they feel gritty; simulated pearls feel smooth. In general, I don't think it's a great idea to rub the pearls your special person has just given you on your teeth as soon as you've opened the gift box. Try to restrain yourself and wait until later. Even if he didn't get you the real thing, he may be real.

Keeping the Sparkle in Your Jewelry

Perfumes and body acids are your jewelry's worst enemies. In addition to periodic checks by jewelers to make sure the prongs that hold stones are not broken or bent, all your jewelry needs a periodic cleaning—not just to make it shine, but to preserve it.

A commercial jewelry cleaner will clean and shine your gold and most stones set in it (not soft stones, such as opals or jade). You can make your own cleaner for gold jewelry that is not set with stones by combining one part ammonia, three parts water, and a few drops of detergent. Clean with a soft brush (old toothbrush) and dry. In between these cleanings, buffing with a soft cloth will help maintain the shine.

Commercial cleaner will clean silver, but if your silver jewelry (without stones) is badly tarnished, you can dip an old toothbrush into a baking soda-and-water paste; brush; rinse; and polish with a soft cloth. For maintenance, buff with a soft cloth between cleanings.

Pearl necklaces (also those of ivory, lapis, jade, coral, and malachite, what I call "soft" stones) need a bath about every sixth time they are worn. Wash in water, to which you've added a few drops of detergent; rinse in clear water; then put a drop or two of mineral oil between your palms and rub the beads gently; let air dry for several hours.

Storage

According to jewelers, the kindest thing you can do for your good jewelry is to store individual pieces in soft flannel or velvet bags—the bags jewelers give you with the jewelry. Makes sense, doesn't it? They give you the bag because it's the best protection for your fine jewelry.

Many people store their opals in water or mixtures of glycerin and water because they say that opals tend to dry out and lose their "fire" after years in the air.

Help! Ring-Finger Emergency

It's horrible to think about, but you can get a ring so stuck on your finger (like when you accidentally smash your finger and it swells) that soaping or oiling or using lotions won't help it slide off.

Try this: get several feet of string; hook about three inches of the string under the ring with the end of the string going toward your palm. You may have to gently push the string through with a match or toothpick if the swelling under the ring is severe. Then, tightly wind the long end of the string around and around your finger, winding it from the ring to your fingernail, and being certain that the string coils are as close to each other as possible, forming a sheath of string on your finger that keeps the swollen tissue from popping through the coils. Holding the coils of string in place as firmly as you can, pull up on the string end that is hooked through your ring, pulling toward the tip of your finger. The coils will unwind as the ring is guided to the end of your finger by the string, which is hooked under the ring. The ring will pop off the end of your finger. It's as if you were unscrewing the ring from your finger along "threads" of string.

Obviously, the sooner you start this trick, the less swelling you'll have to deal with and the less discomfort you will suffer. Should you feel real pain during this procedure, or if your finger becomes discolored or numb, rush to the nearest emergency room or see your doctor as soon as possible.

· DRY CLEANING ·

Too Much Dry Cleaning

Too much dry cleaning does wear out fabrics. It's been estimated that good-quality wool jackets and skirts can survive about five years of regular dry cleaning, but frailer blouses will perish much sooner under such processing. Try to air out and spot-clean outer garments that aren't heavily soiled by perspiration before carting them off to the cleaners. And when you do so, air them out of the sunlight, which is as cruel to colors as it is to your skin. Steaming instead of pressing is kinder to clothing, too. See the section on care labels in Chapter 18, "Let's Go Shopping."

Warnings

Get spotted and stained clothing that can't be laundered to your dry cleaner *as soon as possible* to prevent the stain from setting. Pin a note over the stain telling what it is to make sure it gets noticed and tell the clerk who accepts the garments about the special treatment the garment needs.

Dry Cleaner's Mistakes

It's not always your cleaner's fault. If he is a member of the International Fabricare Institute, they can send the damaged garment to the institute for analysis to determine if damage is the fault of the dry cleaner or the manufacturer or you! If it's the fault of the manufacturer, take the garment back to the store; show a copy of the institute's report, and if you don't get your money back, contact the Better Business Bureau or your local consumer protection agency.

Don't Expect Miracles

Perspiration, water, perfume, and deodorant damage certain fabrics, *especially* silk, so don't blame the cleaner.

Some buttons, sequins, beads, and other decorations may dissolve or be damaged by cleaning fluids. If possible, remove them from the garment before it goes to the cleaner, or take your chances and be graceful when a problem develops.

For best results, take suede or leather to a cleaner who specializes in those materials. Ask your cleaner about leather or suede patches or decorations on clothing before they go into the hopper for cleaning; it may be necessary to send the garments to a special cleaner.

Most people agree that Ultrasuede improves with laundering, getting softer with each washing. Home launder by including towels in the load to fluff up the suede. If your Ultrasuede garment has shoulder pads, take them out. If the lining is unwashable, take it to the cleaner.

Don't dry-clean just the skirt or pants from a suit; have the entire suit cleaned or you may ultimately have a color difference between the two pieces. I know you hate the cost, but it's worth the price—otherwise you may never be able to wear both pieces together.

Judging a Dry Cleaner

Most good dry cleaners are members of the International Fabricare Institute, which provides information on new cleaning techniques, engages in research, and provides the service described in the section of this chapter called "Dry Cleaner's Mistakes."

When you pick up your clothing from the cleaner, it should be bagged properly—not with so many garments in one bag that they are all crushed.

If you are not satisfied with the pressing (which should, by the way, last for several wearings in a good garment), a reputable cleaner will redo the press job; ditto for the cleaning job.

You should not be able to smell cleaning fluid on your clothing; if you can, the solvent is not being filtered properly at the cleaning plant. Don't be afraid to complain.

Good cleaners can do hand pressing and will attach loose buttons and dangling hems without charge. A good dry cleaner is as good a friend as your hairdresser.

Prices

Use the clothing that's not your very best to shop around and test less expensive cleaners. Don't try to save money by using laundromat dry-cleaning machines on clothing that is labeled "professional dry cleaning only" or "commercial dry cleaning only." The money you save will have to be used to buy new garments—"professional" and "commercial" mean just that!

• HOME-LAUNDRY HINTS •

Jeans

I get more questions about why and how the colors of jeans run than there are shades of faded denim.

According to the International Fabricare Institute, the color of new jeans shouldn't run on everything they touch; but this varies with the brand. Repeated prewashing by the manufacturer prevents most running, or "crocking," as the industry calls it, but with all jeans, some crocking is to be expected.

If you want to remove excess dye when it has not been removed by the manufacturer, wash jeans several times before wearing, turning them inside out to prevent streaking, and keeping them separate from the rest of your wash, unless you want a totally blue wardrobe. The institute says there is absolutely nothing that you can add to the water to set the color; all you can do is remove the excess. My readers say they soak them in a salt or vinegar solution and it helps. Couldn't hurt, I say.

Prewash Steps to Take

Before you toss garments into the washer, *read the care label* to be sure they can be laundered, then spot-treat as directed in the section of this chapter on stain removal; brush off excess mud or dirt; brush lint and dirt from pants cuffs; check pockets for items that might damage clothing during the laundry process, such as pens, tissues, or cigarette lighters.

Inside Out

Turn sweaters inside out when laundering to help prevent "pilling" (those little yarn balls that develop on some knit garments). Turning T-shirts that have emblems on them inside out for laundering and drying makes the transfer designs last longer.

Water Temperature

Generally, the hottest water that the fabric can be washed in will give you the whitest, brightest results.

Sorting Wash

If you never listened when your mother told you how to sort the wash, here's how.

Put all whites and light-colored items—bedding, underwear, towels—in one load. White permanent-press and other man-made fabrics tend to act like magnets in picking up color from wash water; always keep them separate from colors.

Delicate knits, sheers, and other similar fabrics that need gentle agitation should be washed together in a separate load. You will find that if you don't load up heavy items like bath towels with delicate items, the delicates will emerge from washing and drying less crushed than they will if they are flattened by heavy pieces in the washer spin cycles and the dryer. Heavy items almost iron in creases in lighter items.

Don't ever wash anything that gives off lots of lint with any dark colors. Dark-colored jeans, corduroys, and other garments pick up lint like pets gather fleas—and the result is about as pleasant!

The time to mix a load is when you're doing sheets. Then it's best to add a few small items, such as pillow cases, underwear, T-shirts, so that the clothing and sheets have space to float around in the washer. They'll get cleaner that way.

Heavily soiled garments should be washed together; if you mix heavily soiled with lightly soiled garments you get instant dingy laundry.

Dingy Laundry

The Heloise never-fail method for getting the dinginess out of laundry is: for bleachable cottons and whites, use a plastic, enamel, or stainless steel container *(never aluminum)*. In it, make a solution of one gallon hot water, one-half cup automatic dishwashing detergent, and one-fourth cup bleach; stir well. Let clothing soak in this solution for thirty minutes. Wash as usual, using one-half cup of white vinegar in the rinse water.

Do not reuse mixture after it has become discolored. Make a fresh batch if you have to do another garment.

When in Doubt

When in doubt, or just on general principles, pull out the instruction booklet that came with your washer and dryer. Manufacturers spend a great deal of money preparing these booklets so that consumers can get the maximum benefit from the appliances they buy. Considering the price of laundry equipment, you owe it to your checkbook to read the booklet, even if you think you understand all of the buttons and dials on your washer and dryer.

Chapter 18

LET'S GO
SHOPPING

· THE BASIC RULES ·

No matter how inexpensive it is, if it doesn't fit right, itches, isn't comfortable, needs a pin somewhere to hold something in place, has a part you feel like tugging on most of the time to keep it where it belongs, is a color that doesn't go with anything else in your wardrobe, makes you feel "not right," needs a major alteration (few garments have enough seam allowance to make them larger), or has a suspicious stain that may not come out, it's *not* a bargain.

This applies to accessories, too. Any part of your wardrobe that spends more of its time in the closet or dresser drawer than on you is not really a part of your wardrobe—and that includes those cute shoes that you bought on sale, thinking they'd fit "when they stretch out." Shoes that hurt your feet don't usually get stretched out because you don't wear them. They are like the purses that are supposed to "go with everything" and really go only with a closet shelf, or the necklaces that look good in a department store's velvet showcase, but are the wrong length for any of your clothes and spend most of their time in your jewelry box.

• *WHEN TO SHOP* •

You'll get the best selection when the seasonal merchandise has just arrived, the best buys off-season. Generally, spring merchandise starts arriving in February, hits its peak in March, and sales on the first arrivals begin in April. You'll get the best selection of summer clothes in May. July sales follow the inventory period, and by the end of July fall clothing is beginning to show up in stores. The best selection time for fall clothing is at the end of July or in August. October and November features dressy holiday clothing, and resort wear arrives in December and January. Sales that clear out seasonal merchandise are great for finding what you need, not just items you want. See "Learning to Speak Sale Language" in this chapter for schedules.

• *WHEN NOT TO SHOP* •

Shop when the stores are the least crowded; mornings and during the dinner hour are best. In certain areas of the country, many people go to church services on Wednesday evening. And a major sporting or festival event will draw crowds away from stores or keep people in front of their TV sets on a certain night. This is especially true toward the end of football season when the important games are on TV. In San Antonio, a certain wallpaper store is always open on Sunday afternoons. Why? The store's clerks say that football widows get their revenge on their TV-mesmerized husbands by picking out great quantities of wallpaper for their "sports" to put up after the game is over. Now, don't think I'm recommending such revenge—I'm a football fan myself! But it *is* a thought . . .

Don't shop when you are depressed. If you need to buy yourself a little present for an emotional lift—and most of us do every now and then—shop at a thrift shop or another place where you won't be tempted to spend a lot of money on something you'll never wear when you are feeling like your old self again.

Also, don't shop when you look bad, like after you've had a tooth pulled at the dentist's, or on that magic day when your hair suddenly becomes one inch too long and your hairstyle is totally out of shape. If you shop when you look bad, you aren't likely to find anything that looks good on you.

If you are dress shopping, you'll make better judgments if you wear pantyhose and a slip—unless, of course, you can use your imagination when you are trying on a dress while wearing knee-highs or socks with clunky walking shoes or sneakers. Also, if you shop at discount stores and have to try on clothing in one of those community dressing rooms, you won't feel as self-conscious when you strip to fit. Many women prefer to wear a full slip or a leotard when they go bargain hunting.

And, of course, don't shop for shoes at the end of your shopping trip. Your feet are likely to be swollen and you'll buy yourself a pair of gunboats that you can only wear with athletic socks—not such a hot idea if they're satin cocktail party shoes. Shoe shopping with puffy feet may not be a totally bad idea if you are actually looking for shoes that you'll be walking in for hours, such as tourist shoes. Perhaps you should buy walking shoes midway through your shopping trek.

• WHERE TO SHOP •

Don't restrict yourself to ladies, women's, or juniors departments. Small women especially can find great bargains in children's clothing, which is generally made for endurance and, these days, is modeled after adult fashions. You can find underwear, nightgowns, robes, sportswear, summer jewelry, and all sorts of accessories. (Junior sizes go up to thirteen.) Go to the boys department to find sportswear, jackets, vests, sweaters, and shirts. Same goes for the men's department; you can find shirts, sweaters, and accessories such as ascots, ties, and some belts, as well as the usual unisex jeans.

And while you're shopping, don't forget that many lingerie garments can double for evening wear—and save you money.

And not all the bargains are at resale shops, thrift stores, or discount houses; you can find jackets, web belts for sportswear, backpacks to take shopping (instead of toting everything on your arm), luggage or tote bags, and many fun sportswear garments at your local army surplus store.

Here's another idea: if you usually wear functional, sturdy underwear, but like to have a few frivolous, lacy bras and panties when you feel frivolous and lacy, try the dime store. Undies that don't get washed and dried in machines every week don't need to be durable. The same thing goes for lacy blouses or evening wear: they don't get worn and laundered as often as your everyday clothes, so they can be delicate.

• *CATALOG SHOPPING* •

This is becoming increasingly popular with women whose working hours make store shopping difficult. Be sure to check the measurement guide in the book before determining sizes. In the most popular catalogs, you'll find "good, better, best" categories, and this is helpful in choosing quality.

It's important to keep copies or at least records of what you have ordered. Time passes quickly and we do forget. In fact, it's important to *always* keep your receipts, whether you shop in catalogs or stores. Often a defect will show up after the garment is laundered or dry-cleaned, or the dry cleaner will damage a garment, and having a receipt is the best proof of price. Receipts are especially important if you pay cash—whether it's at a catalog pick-up or in a department store. If you need to return a receipt with a catalog order, be sure to keep a copy—the few pennies it costs to use a copier are worth it.

• *LEARNING TO SPEAK SALE LANGUAGE* •

We all know that regular merchandise gets marked down to make room for new stock, but here are some other common terms.

Clearance Sale

Check these items carefully. They are being "cleared" because they have been in stock too long; they may be shop-worn and are sold "as is," usually with no return.

Comparable Value

In the store's opinion, the item they are selling for $12.95 compares in value to a similar item sold in other stores for $24.95. Your opinion may not be the same as the store's, so check out the competition.

Irregulars

Inspect them carefully to find out what's irregular about them. They can be a good buy if they are wearable. I've seen shirts marked irregular that seem to have a longer shirttail or sleeve than shirts of comparable size; this can actually be an advantage.

Liquidation Sale

This is supposed to mean that the store is going out of business, but sometimes certain stores seem to use "going out of business" as a sales trap, even if some states have laws restricting the number of going-out-of-business sales a store can have.

Special Purchase

The store got a bargain from a manufacturer who couldn't sell the merchandise at its regular price, and it's passing that bargain on to you.

Event Sales

Store birthdays or anniversaries may offer bargains, especially among "loss leader" items marked way down to lure you into the store and tempt you to buy other things at regular prices.

Holiday Sales

In most parts of the country, you'll find major mark-down periods after Christmas, Easter, after or on July 4, Columbus Day, Washington's Birthday. In some parts of the country, sales will be held in conjunction with local celebrations.

Monthly Specials

Certain items get marked down in most parts of the country on a predictable monthly schedule. Here are the months and the usual sales and wardrobe items:

• *January:* after-Christmas clearances and preinventory sales, costume jewelry, furs, lingerie, pocket books, shoes
• *February:* men's clothing, sports apparel and equipment
• *March:* boy's and girl's shoes, infants' clothing, ice skates and ski equipment, luggage
• *April:* fabrics, hosiery, lingerie, women's shoes
• *May:* handbags, housecoats, jewelry, luggage, shoes, sportswear, Mothers' Day specials
• *June:* fabrics, lingerie, sleepwear and hosiery, men's clothing and Fathers' Day specials, women's shoes
• *July:* bathing suits, children's clothing, handbags, lingerie and sleepwear, luggage, men's shirts and shoes, sportswear, summer clothes
• *August:* back-to-school specials, bathing suits, cosmetics, furs, men's coats, women's coats
• *September:* fabrics, fall fashions
• *October:* fall and winter clothing, lingerie and hosiery, women's coats, other storewide clearances
• *November:* boys' suits and coats, lingerie, men's suits and coats, shoes, winter clothing
• *December:* children's clothes, coats and hats, men's furnishings, resort and cruise wear, shoes

• *INSIDES AND OUTSIDES OF BUYING FOR QUALITY* •

When you are looking for quality, clothing is like people—much of what's good or bad doesn't show up at first glance, and some defects that at first seem tolerable will cause problems later on.

Here are some ways to check for quality in garments.

Buttons, Buttonholes, and Zippers

Do the buttons add or detract from the look of the garment? Are they all on, and/or is there a spare? Can they be replaced if lost, or if you just don't like them? Buttons that will look better longer are those made from mother-of-pearl, wood, or bone instead of plastic. Are the buttonholes frayed? Are they placed properly so the garment doesn't gap in strange places, such as those that leave a bustline gap on your dress or blouse?

Do the zippers jam? Are they the right color? (Especially check color on irregular garments.) Is the zipper set properly or is there a gap at either end of the zipper? Is the stitching straight, or does the zipper pucker from improper stitching?

Cut

Whether a garment part is cut on the straight or bias (crosswise) of the fabric determines how it will keep its shape. Occasionally, you'll see a garment part not cut exactly on the straight or exactly crosswise/bias, and it is obviously not how the designer intended the fabric to be cut. After washing or dry cleaning, such defects in the cut will prevent the garment from hanging properly, even if the garment looked all right when new.

Fabric

Crush it in your hand. Does it wrinkle easily? Even with new techniques pure linens and cottons wrinkle. This wrinkle is sort of in with some people who like the natural look, but if you feel uncomfortable with wrinkles, better choose combinations of natural and man-made fibers that won't get them. Most people agree that the greater the percentage of natural fiber—cotton, silk, linen, wool—the more comfortable the garment will feel when worn.

Look for imperfections in the fabric. Some fabrics have slubs and irregular woven thread patterns as part of their character; others may just snag easily or have defects.

Color

If the garment has matching pieces, check to make sure they really do match; garments from different dye lots may not match exactly, and the lighting in some stores is deceptive and may change color tones. I now own a purple silk dress that I thought was blue! I still wear it, but my blue shoes sure don't go with it.

Collars

If there is topstitching, is it even? Are there puckers or irregular folds at the seam line? Does the collar lay properly? If the clerk says a pressing will solve any problem that you notice, ask the clerk to press it to make sure. Are both top and underside of the collar of the same fabric and cut? Checking collars is especially important when buying irregulars. I have seen collars that were actually off-center! You could never wear such a garment.

Linings

Does the color match or complement the garment? Is the lining set properly so it won't bind or hang out from the bottom or sleeve hems? In a good jacket or coat, you will find about one-quarter to one-half an inch folded on the sleeve and bottom hems to allow for your movement inside the garment; this prevents the lining from tearing when you reach for something or sit down. Skirt linings are not attached to the hems, except sometimes at certain points if they need to be anchored.

Pants

These can be taken in on the back seam and legs for a better fit, but if they don't fit properly in the hips or crotch when you bend or sit, it's unlikely that there will be enough seam allowance to let out for a fit.

When you try on pants, wear the shoes you will wear with the pants so that you can check the length. Sometimes pants can be shortened, but if they are tapered, it's unlikely that you will have the right shape and tapered look once you have shortened the leg. If the leg is perfectly straight, you may be able to lengthen or shorten it without too much trouble. In some pants, the fabric may have been pressed too firmly. You may have a problem getting rid of the crease, even if you dab the hem with vinegar before pressing, which works on some fabrics. (Yes, I know, vinegar again!) My advice is to look for proportioned pants that don't need adjustment in the leg.

If you have a lot of problems finding pants that fit, you may want to have your slacks made at a tailor—well-fitted pants will get worn enough to justify the investment, and a tailor or seamstress will keep your measurements for repeat orders. The alternative is to sew them yourself. Many sewing centers—those that give lessons and sell machines—have special courses in which you design a master pattern tailored to your measurements that you can use over and over again, forever banishing the miseries of poorly fitted pants.

Pockets

Are they set well? Do they show through the garment because they are too bulky? Are patch pockets sewn without puckers, with even curves or angles?

Prints and Plaids

The patterns of prints and plaids should match; if they don't (and sometimes a style prevents matching at all seams), does the non-match take away from the overall look of the garment? Nonwoven prints or plaids—those that have been imprinted on the fabric— should especially be checked for flaws in the pattern. You can tell if a pattern is imprinted or woven by checking the inside; naturally, printed patterns don't go all the way through.

Seams

Do they pucker? Are they straight or curved, as they should be? Does the thread match or at least not mismatch? Are there threads hanging from seams and topstitching, and will the garment become a clown's break-away suit if you pull one of these threads? Again, if the clerk tells you all a bad seam needs is pressing, ask to have it pressed to make sure; unless you don't mind resewing a garment.

Few garments have enough of a seam allowance to let out, so don't buy a too-small garment without checking the seams first.

Shoulder Pads

Are they properly set and shaped? If a garment is washable, are the shoulder pads also washable, or will they mat or lose their shape? You can put pads in almost any garment to help change the line and give it a more finished and expensive look.

Skirts and Dresses

Look for hems deep enough to be lowered when fashion dictates longer skirts, unless you ignore changing skirt lengths. And remember, if a skirt has a border design on it, you can forget any lengthening or shortening plans unless the border doesn't matter, and I can't imagine that. If a skirt has a slit, make sure one side of the opening is not longer than the other.

• *CARE LABELS* •

Make sure care labels are on the garment. You also need to check out fabrics that may irritate your skin. If a garment can only be dry-cleaned, decide if you want to pay for dry cleaning—especially in a garment that will be frequently worn and cleaned.

Here are some of the new (as of January 1, 1984) government regulations on care labels to make life easier for you when you are deciding on laundering and dry-cleaning methods for your clothing.

Wash or Dry-Clean

Labels must say whether a garment should be washed or dry-cleaned, and if both methods can be used, the manufacturers can choose to give instructions for either method or instructions for both on the label.

Dry-Cleaning Instructions

When dry cleaning is recommended on the label, the manufacturer must include the name of at least one type of solvent that can be used. An example: "professionally dry-clean—fluorocarbon." If any commercially available solvent can be used on the garment, the label need not list the name of a solvent.

Machine- or Hand-Wash

Labels must specify whether a garment is to be washed by hand or machine and tell the proper water temperature. Water temperature does not need to be mentioned if using hot water regularly will not damage the garment. If the label says "machine-wash" it means hot, warm, or cold water can be used.

Bleach

If regular use of bleach will harm the garment, words or a phrase to indicate this, such as, "do not bleach," must be on the label. If any kind of bleach can be used, the label doesn't have to mention bleaching. If any bleach but chlorine bleach can be used, the label must say "only nonchlorine bleach, when needed."

Machine- or Line-Dry

The drying method must be indicated on labels. If the garment is to be machine-dried, the drying temperature must be specified, unless the highest heat setting on a dryer won't harm the garment.

Ironing

If regular ironing is not required, no instructions need be given. If regular ironing is required, instructions must be given, along with recommendations for the temperature to be used. If regular use of a hot iron won't harm the item, no instructions are required.

Warnings

If any part of the label's washing or dry-cleaning instructions could harm the garment, or others being cleaned with it, there must be a clearly worded warning, such as: "do not," "no," "only," accompanied by instructions. For example, a label might warn: "do not iron" or "professionally dry-clean, no steam."

Exemptions from Permanent Care Labels

Only garments that can be cleaned safely with the harshest methods are exempt from requiring permanent care labels, but even then, the garment's tag or package must state, "wash or dry-clean, any normal method," so you won't have to guess.

• GENERAL SHOPPING HINTS •

Some folks love to shop, others think it's just one more chore. Here are some hints from my readers, plus some of my own tips for saving money, simplifying shopping, and avoiding all those headache-making decisions that take all the fun out of adding to and updating a wardrobe.

Bargain Hunting

Don't forget thrift shops and rummage sales for bargains. You can profit from someone else's mistakes and look great in their bad buys.

And don't be afraid to ask for discounts on buttonless, damaged, but fixable garments—even if they already have been marked down.

At some stores, you'll find merchandise that's been returned and stashed in the back room, where you can buy it at discount. Other stores authorize clerks to give away extras to customers who make large purchases—a scarf, belt, or other accessory to go with one of those dresses you just bought. Ask. Don't be embarrassed. They can only say no; but they just might say yes and make your day.

Color Scheming

A garment in the hand is worth two in the mind's eye. If you are trying to match a color (or texture), such as a blouse to a suit or a belt to a dress, wear the garment or just take a part of it—the skirt or vest—with you when you go shopping. Not even all blacks and whites always match, so the possibility of your picking the right color *without* a swatch is slim. I have seven different black skirts, jackets, and blazers, and some of them look tacky if I try to put them together.

Great Reruns

Keep lists or remember, if you can, which stores and manufacturers have clothing that best fits and flatters your proportions. This saves time and energy. And isn't fit always a problem, especially jeans and slacks, until you hit on the manufacturer who seems to have you in mind? Once you get a brand name and style that fits, stick with it. So what if you have the same slacks in three colors? How many hours of my life have been wasted trying on what seems like hundreds of size tens and finding only three that fit!

How Much Is Too Much?

You figure out your food budget per serving, right? Well, it works the same with clothing. How often will you wear that $250 suit or that $100 dress? Once a month? Rarely? Twice a week? Can the jacket and skirt mix and match with other parts of your wardrobe? The $250 suit could be a real bargain because you'll wear it often, whereas the $100 dress winds up a bad buy because you can only wear it to weddings or the Christmas party. How often can you wear the dress if you travel with the same crowd? Never, never buy anything just because it's cheap. Unless that markdown item is beautifully basic or can be worn with clothing you already have, or you really love it, you'll just be acquiring another closet stuffer.

There are, of course, exceptions to every rule. I once found a designer blouse on sale for $10 (marked down from $100). I wear it when I repot plants because the color is a shade of green that I don't like; but in my $100 blouse I feel chic, so why not?

Pressure Buying

Don't do it! Don't ever race through the stores on Saturday morning looking for something—anything—to wear on Saturday night. You'll end up with a closet stuffer that probably costs twice as much as you can afford. And while we're on the subject of pressure buying, look out for sales clerks who flatter you, friends who really want that puce chiffon cocktail dress for themselves, and (just between us) look out for your mom, who always picks out blouses that look better on your cousin. Learn how to say, "Yes, you're right, but that's not right for me" . . . nicely.

What's on First?

Buy the hardest thing to find first. For example, buy your print blouse and then look for coordinating pants or skirt. But if you have fitting problems with pants or skirts, then buy the hard-to-fit parts first and the coordinating blouses, belts, and accessories afterward.

Chapter 19

ON THE ROAD

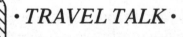

· TRAVEL TALK ·

Let's see. Where to begin? Should I start by telling you how friendly everyone is just about everywhere I go? Do I rhapsodize about the delicious food here, there, and everywhere? Do I tell you about the beautiful sights and countryside I've seen?

I'd need more space than there is in this book to share my travel joys. So I think I'll stick to what I've learned about the practical side of traveling—the challenge of packing everything I'll need for two weeks in one bag and one carry-on garment hang-up bag, for example.

I travel a lot more than most people imagine. And I love it—not only because seeing new sights is fun, but because it enables me to meet the people who read my columns and books. Over the years, I have learned—often by trial and error—how to travel as efficiently as possible, with the least amount of fuss and trauma. And I'm still learning!

Planning a trip can be half of the fun, and if you rely on a good travel agent, it will be pretty painless. Did you know that travel agencies don't cost you extra? You can ask them to make your plans and hotel reservations, check prices, all for free. Agents know the up-to-the-minute prices and money-exchange rates (if you are going out of the country). They keep track of changes in air schedules, so they can get you where you are going in the easiest, fastest, and least expensive way. Very often a travel agent has already been to your destination and can tell you how to get to the hotel from the airport, how long it will take, and what it will cost. They can tell you about the hotel, suggest places to eat, any other attractions, and so forth.

How do you find a travel agent? Ask friends who travel frequently to recommend one. Visit or call the agency and ask about their services. Will they deliver tickets? Can they make *all* of your plans?

Once you establish a working relationship with your travel agency, and the agent knows your needs and preferences, all the travel planning that you could waste a lot of time on will be done for you. I used to spend a lot of time making air reservations. No longer—because my travel agent Linda does it all! Nowadays agencies use computers that can come up with the information you want in a matter of seconds.

Let's say your plans are made. The next step is to decide what to take with you. How many changes of clothing are you *really* going to need? Contrary to what your mother may have told you, if you will be going to several different places, and seeing different people, you don't need a change of clothes for each day. Take it from me— nobody is going to point at you and say, "That woman has on the same blouse that she wore four days ago." And if someone does, tough!

Think about the types of clothing you'll require. Are you going to the beach? Do you need warm clothes? Do you need dressy clothes? Or can you get by with slacks, T-shirts, and shorts? Then, think about what you really *want* to take, and write it all down. These few minutes will save you much time and trouble later on. I promise.

For example, I usually plan it so that I can wear the dress I wore Monday night again on Friday or Saturday, with a little jacket and a different belt or different-colored stockings. After you've written it all down, go over your list and ask yourself if you really and truly need everything on it. You'll find that most of the time, you don't need to take as much as you anticipate—especially if you adopt some of my travel and packing tips.

When I told a friend of mine that I was going to Europe for seventeen days and did not plan to check any luggage at the airport, she didn't believe me. But I did exactly as I said and showed her my packing system to prove it (described later in this chapter).

Believe me, packing for a trip, even for a two-week trip, doesn't necessarily require much pain and suffering. Make a "grocery" list of what you'll need, then add the extras.

The real secret to a travel wardrobe is to go with one color scheme. Personally, I like dear old basic black—it goes well with gray, white, red, and sometimes blue. When I want a change, I use gray, red, blue, and add a touch of burgundy or black.

A mix-and-match wardrobe really is simple once you get the hang of it. That's why it's vital to write everything down, so you can see at a glance what you can mix with what. You don't want to end up on the road with a pink blouse that really doesn't go with anything. And as a rule of thumb it's a good idea to avoid bringing anything that only can be worn once—unless it's a formal gown for an important special event.

White and black are two basic colors that are always safe and versatile.

Here's my traveling wardrobe:

- One black suit
- One gray skirt (can be of the same material as the black skirt)
- Coordinating blazer, jacket, or vest
- Three blouses in white, red, and gray, or a print consisting of these colors
- Pullover, turtleneck, or other sweater (for cool weather)
- A couple of belts—gold, black, and/or gray
- One extra pair of walking shoes

Add for evening:

- Black dressy slacks
- Overshirt of similar fabric in black or white
- Camisole or tube top

For evening wear, I like to have a pair of black dressy slacks and team them with an overshirt of similar fabric, and maybe wear a camisole or tube top under the shirt, and then add an accent belt. For a casual, chic look, I pull up my shirt collars, roll up the shirt sleeves, and wear comfortable sandals. All of these are comfortable and pack well.

When you're planning your wardrobe, make sure that your fabrics go well together so that even though you are mixing and matching, it doesn't look like it. Most people prefer to take solid or subtly patterned clothing because you can get bored with your own clothing if you have to wear a busy print dress too often. Try to limit your colors and patterns to blouses and scarves.

Of course, shoes and handbags must coordinate with your outfits, but remember, in the evening you can cheat a little—black and dark navy look the same under night lights. Also for evening, a small lightweight evening bag is a good choice.

My favorite pair of traveling shoes are gray and black—they go with almost everything I wear. I always have several extra pairs of hose in matching colors, a slip, nightgown, and cover-up. And of course I add makeup, vitamins, prescriptions, and grooming items.

When you think of something that you need to take, write it down on your list or go get it and throw it into the suitcase. I usually start packing about three or four days before I go on a trip. I put my suitcase out and just plop things in when I think about them. There are times when I'm traveling so much that the suitcase stays on my bathroom floor—packed or repacked with toiletries and makeup.

Here was my "must list" for my Europe trip. My clothing included basics, such as one fancy black dress, black slacks and blazer, along with a few colored shirts, bright scarves, and feminine-style ties—all of which were great because they were very light and didn't take up much space in the suitcase I carried around for two weeks. I also included a list of the mix-and-match possibilities I had planned and attached it to the garment's hanger for reference. (Some people do this for their everyday clothing as well as for travel wardrobes. This list or menu is a must when I'm on a public relations tour.)

My basic list of creature comforts includes: makeup, hair-care items, body-care items, and any medication. Remember, always save or buy the little sample sizes of shampoo, creme rinse, etc. I have even found sample sizes of nasal spray no bigger than your thumb (if your thumb isn't too small).

In a pinch, shampoo can double as laundry soap, and cream rinse can double as shaving cream. The trick is to make sure that everything, and I do mean *everything*, is as small and light as possible. And don't carry glass—it's too heavy.

Here's a simple list of necessary items:

• Brush, comb, curlers, other hair aids
• Toothbrush, toothpaste (save the smidgens at the end of a big tube for travel)
• Shaving equipment
• Bath powder, deodorant, perfume
• Cotton balls/swabs
• Makeup
• Eyeglasses and/or contacts (and an extra pair)
• Credit cards, traveler's checks, "tip money"—single dollars or loose change
• Small notebook and pen (to keep track of phone numbers, expenses, people's names)
• Don't forget your tickets!

I keep a permanent set of toiletries and a traveling makeup kit in my bag so that I don't have to pack and repack my cosmetics. If you keep a travel makeup kit and travel often, don't forget to replenish supplies after your return, while you still remember what you used up. It saves last-minute rushes.

One thing I have done when traveling that really cuts down on weight and space is to find out if the hotel I'm headed for provides hair dryers. Some even have electric razors and curlers available on request. If you can find the hotel's 800 phone number, it won't cost you anything to call them and ask, and you may be surprised at the many services available to guests. If you plan to use their iron and ironing board to press your own clothing, do find out beforehand if you're going to be charged for it. Some hotels provide them at no charge and others charge so much that it's almost cheaper to go out and buy these things and leave them behind! A friend of mine was billed $20 for use of an ironing board in an East Coast hotel. She couldn't believe it. I can't either.

You probably are asking yourself how you are going to fit everything into those carry-on bags. I'll admit that this trick almost takes as much luck and skill as fitting a size eight and a half foot into a size seven sale shoe. But it is possible. I promise.

First, don't wait until two hours before your flight to pack. I seem to get better about packing things as my trip wears on, so practice

—you may be surprised to find that you will have a little more room than expected.

Remember, heavy things go on the bottom of your suitcase (or what will be the bottom when it is picked up and carried). You don't want to pick up the suitcase and then have everything slide down to the bottom and squish your lightweight things. When you put shoes in a regular suitcase, put them sole to sole, with the heel of one shoe touching the toe of the other. Stuff small, light things into them so that they keep their shape. I stuff shoes with pantyhose, slips, even pill bottles and bags of vitamins.

Fill out the empty spaces with soft things, such as socks and underwear or T-shirts. Put large clothing items on the top. Skirts should go in flat and fold once; pants can be matched cuff to cuff and then folded in half or rolled up. To pack a dress, hold it up by the shoulders, place it in the suitcase so that the top of the dress is in the suitcase and the skirt is draped over the edge. Then fold the sleeves across the front of the dress, and fold the skirt up across the dress top. If the skirt is very full, fold the sides inward first, and then fold up the skirt. Stuff tissue or underwear into the folds of clothing to prevent creases. Make sure all clothing is buttoned, zipped, and belted to keep its shape. I carry a hanging garment bag so that I don't have to fold skirts, blouses, and dresses.

Some people put slacks or seldom-used items on the bottom, shirts and nightclothes on top, underwear on one side and cosmetics on the other, heavy shoes at the back (which becomes the bottom when the suitcase is picked up). Then, they put appliances, such as hair dryers and irons, in the middle.

But each of us has to pack according to what works for us. You don't want to unload everything every day to get at things on the bottom. The key here is finding the system that works for you. If things are always put where they belong, you are less likely to lose them in your travels.

No packing advice would be complete without unpacking advice. Well, my advice is, when the time comes to unpack, don't. Unless you are going to be in one place for a few days, it really is easier to pull out only the things you need. This way it's much easier to repack when it's time to move on.

But I have a confession. I only do the above—don't unpack all the way—once in a while. Usually, if I am making more than a one-night stand, I hang things up, pull out my makeup, set things on the desk and elsewhere. I think I do this because I travel so much, and it's important for me to try to make the hotel room seem like home, or at least comfortable and a little familiar. Somehow seeing *my* clock next to the bed, and *my* paper work on the desk makes the room seem a little cozier.

Being comfortable when you travel is vital to making sure your trip becomes a fond memory. A well-planned wardrobe, efficient packing, and well-organized travel details are the surest way to eliminate the stresses and strains that keep you from looking and feeling your beautiful best on the road.

• TAKE-ALONGS •

In my travels, I've learned that little things can add up to big conveniences. A little know-how helps to ease the pain and strain of making do with what's available when you're checked into a home away from home.

For example, if you pack a couple of plastic clothespins, you'll be able to fasten your skirts to an ordinary hanger if the hotel hasn't provided skirt hangers; or keep your swimsuit, undies, or pantyhose from slipping off whatever you've hung them on to dry inside the shower (they won't dry if they spend the night crumpled in the bottom of the tub).

You can use your clothespins to position wet things near the heating or air-conditioning vents in your hotel room for better air drying, or to keep that bikini drying on the balcony from blowing down to the street. (If you forget the pins, sometimes you can weave a garment into the plastic webbing of balcony chairs, but make sure you're discreet about it.)

The best solution is to try to avoid laundry on a long trip by traveling with disposables. In a pinch, you can make disposable panties from pantyhose by cutting off the legs after they've gone to runs.

Here are some other take-alongs to make your traveling more pleasant.

Extras

If you're a dedicated shopper, or even if you're not, packing an extra cloth folding suitcase—especially on vacation—will prevent you from overloading your luggage with souvenirs you purchase along the way. There are so many temptations to buy when traveling. A friend of mine's motto is: "If you don't like it, just buy two."

Food Fix

If you are the kind who gets limp or cranky when your meal schedule is upset by changing time zones, pack a few crackers or some dried fruit or nuts to soothe those out-of-step hunger pangs.

Light

A purse-size flashlight or a small plug-in nightlight can come in handy, especially in a strange room when you are fumbling around in the dark for a light switch. Some travelers who get disoriented in hotel rooms leave the bathroom light on overnight—just a crack of light from the door helps you remember if it's Tuesday and if it's Belgium.

Lost and Found

Take a matchbook from each motel or hotel you visit so you'll know where your home away from home is. This comes in very handy when you're coming back after a party and the taxi driver never heard of the place! You'll have the name and address handy later on, if you leave something behind when you check out. Also, tape your name and address *inside* your luggage in case your luggage tags get ripped off and your luggage takes off on a trip of its own.

Always hang on to your luggage check-in receipts, and if your luggage gets lost, report it *immediately*.

Mail-outs

Since carrying around brochures and souvenirs will eventually weigh you down, take along self-addressed manila envelopes and mailing labels, along with a large envelope or wrapping paper and tape, so that you can just post these things home to yourself.

Passport

As soon as you know that you are going to a foreign country other than Canada and Mexico (where your voter registration card is acceptable as proof of citizenship), apply for a passport; it takes several weeks to receive it after application. It's good for ten years now, and costs $35, plus a $7 execution fee. If you've had a passport before, you may be able to renew it by mail; otherwise, head for a federal or state court or a post office that can give you the necessary forms and instructions you need to get passports.

Plastic Bags

Take along extralarge plastic bags to hold the laundry that didn't get quite dry before you moved on, to hold your shoes so that they won't get your other clothing dirty, or to protect your camera in the rain. A larger bag can be an emergency rain hat. It may look silly, but after the rain, your hair will be drier than the hair of folks who got wet because they weren't as creative as you were. For more on plastic bags, see the general hints section.

Sleep

If you're a very light sleeper, toss in earplugs and a sleep mask to keep out the dawn, so that you can make your own dark, quiet refuge wherever you go. Earplugs are a must for me.

Soap

Carry along the soap your skin is used to if you have any skin problems, and save the motel/hotel soap bars to carry in your purse for use at service station stops, where soap is often a rare find. Yes, I take home pretty soap bars; I haven't bought soap in years!

Sponge

Most hotels provide washcloths, but I pack a quick-drying foam bath sponge because I like it better than a washcloth and it doesn't add any weight.

Tie-ups

A small roll of masking tape, a small ball of twine, and one of those stretchable cords—the kind with hooks on both ends that kids often use to hold books on bike carriers—will keep you put together in case your suitcase needs help staying closed or anything else comes apart.

Toter

To carry your luggage on the plane, get a good collapsible luggage cart—that is, unless you've been in a weight-lifting program. Don't buy lightweight quality—it won't last if you travel a lot.

Tummy Helpers

Many a trip is ruined by tummy upsets caused by changes in routine, food, etc. One help is the new "yogurt in a pill," an acidophilus pill, which will help you maintain the right combination of bacteria in your intestines, thereby avoiding digestive upsets. An antacid is also a good addition to your personal first-aid kit. And, of course, don't forget any medication you normally take and a written prescription if you're on a long foreign trip. Remember, also, to pack an extra pair of eyeglasses and/or contacts.

Umbrella

If you don't have a fold-up, lightweight rain cap, make one with a one-yard square of plastic—such as the plastic from a paint drop cloth. Cut a face-size hole in the middle. Fold it up to the size of the plastic sandwich bag you'll stash it in, and—voilà!—you have an umbrella and rain cap/coat that weighs almost nothing. You won't be a fashion plate, but you will be dry. You can also use the plastic square as a cushion for when you pause to rest during tours. (Getting the back of your coat, skirt, or slacks muddy or dirty can dampen your enthusiasm for even the most scenic of sights.)

Weather

Check out the weather at your destination so you can be prepared whether it's with a sweater or coat, a sundress or a shawl.

· *GENERAL HINTS* ·

Airline Seating

For the smoothest ride, get seats in the middle compartment over the wing's forward part. For the quietest ride, go to the front section. You'll get the most leg room in seats around the exits or at bulkheads, and in the first rows of each section. Seats in the last section don't always fully recline. Aisle seats provide more elbow room.

If you are a nonsmoker, be sure to sit at least five rows ahead of the smoking section. I know that in some countries nonsmoking is on side-by-side halves of the plane; check on this before you book reservations, especially if you really can't tolerate smoke.

If you don't want to see the movie, you may want to sit directly beneath the screen because this is where you get extra leg room.

Addresses

Whenever traveling, always have your staying address on your person. Your driver's license with your address back home is not going to help the police find the relatives waiting for you at their home or in the hotel if something should happen to you.

Attachments

Men and women who wear ties can clip tie bars or stick pins to the ties they'll be worn with. This way there's no chance of losing them. Brooches can be attached to the garment they'll be worn with also.

Bags

You can make your own toiletry kit, laundry or shoe bag from the good parts of an old shower curtain, or you can buy a new curtain or liner and make yourself a matching set of bags.

To make a laundry or shoe bag, the trick is to work with the top of the shower curtain where the grommet holes for hanging it are located. Cut two pieces, fourteen by eighteen inches, rounding the corners opposite the grommet holes. Stitch bag sections together, leaving the top grommeted edges open. For a decorative touch, cover the seam edges by stitching on double-fold bias tape. Make drawstrings to thread through the grommet holes by stitching the double-fold bias tape closed. Thread through the grommets and tie in a bow to close the top.

To make a toiletry kit, cut two pieces, eight by fourteen and a half inches, and one piece sixteen by fourteen and a half inches. Trim the long sides of the two smaller pieces with bias tape. Then place the smaller pieces on the larger piece, meeting the trimmed edges in the center. Cut the outer corners into a smooth curve (you can use a saucer to get the curve outline). Then enclose the entire edge of the kit with bias tape. Then cut two pieces of tape to serve as ties and to use on the stitching line that will form pockets. Place these bias strips on the outside of the case, so that they form three equal sections, and stitch all three layers as well as the ends of the tape. Fold over your compartmented bag and tie shut.

For either bag, you can use a fancy, decorative machine stitch on the bias before you sew it on for an extra touch.

Cameras

Don't lose your camera! Before packing your camera and film, put your address sticker on your camera and its removable parts, such as removable flash, and then put transparent tape over the label. Your camera and its parts can be returned to you if you leave them behind. If you are concerned about someone knowing your home address, put your phone number or your work address on a label.

Cardboard Tubes

If longer dresses drag on the floor of your car, or get crumpled up on the bottom of your carry-on hanging bag, slit a cardboard tube and put it over the hanger. Then you can fold your dress at the waist over the cardboard tube and it will only be half as long. This way it won't get dirty or crushed either.

Slippery fabrics can be held in place with spring clothespins. In fact, just about anything can be held in place with spring clothespins. I prefer the new plastic-covered metal clothespins you can buy by the bag in variety stores.

Check! Check!

If you do check luggage on a plane, make sure the clerk puts the correct destination on the tags. Luggage can get sidetracked if your tag mistakenly shows one of the plane stops as the final destination. That's one reason I always carry on my baggage!

Coffee Breaks

If you have the space (and you probably want to make space), pack a hot pot or little portable heater to heat water for your morning coffee or afternoon tea. Then you can have instant room service whenever you want it without inflated prices and tipping. Who needs to wait forty-five minutes for coffee that may arrive lukewarm! And, oh, I love having my morning coffee while I dress, or putting my feet up and settling down with a nice hot drink after a full day. You can collect the extra instant decaf coffee packets some restaurants and hotels serve or just buy samples of instant coffee when available. Another trick is to measure out the coffee, creamer, and sweetener into plastic bags. And for other travel treats, don't forget instant cocoa packets and spiced cider powder packs— they're cheap and convenient.

Customs

When you travel overseas, make sure you can bring your souvenirs home *before* you spend your hard-earned money buying them. You may have trouble transporting fresh fruits and other foods; different states/ports of entry in the United States have different laws concerning importing liquor. And don't try to fool customs officials; they have information on what items are made in the USA and those made in foreign countries.

Ask about duty-free items; items bought from developing countries may be duty-free.

Diet Food

If you're on a special diet of vegetarian, allergy, kosher, or low-cal foods, place a special order when you make your plane reservations.

Avoid overindulging in alcohol and food to prevent that overstuffed, overeverything feeling you can get when cooped up in a plane for so many hours. Some people avoid caffeine, too.

Dirty Laundry

Most hotels furnish laundry bags for guests to use when sending out laundry. You can use these bags for take-home laundry. Or you can carry along an old pillowcase for dirty laundry. Just remember to fold up dirty laundry so it fits into your suitcase the way it did when it was clean—bunched up laundry seldom fits anywhere but the trunk of a car.

Drying Up and Out

Before you hang up your drip-dry wash, roll it in a towel to squeeze out as much moisture as you can; then blow it dry with your hair dryer if you are in a hurry.

Eating on a Budget

Room service menus are usually higher than dining room service and there's always a surcharge and a tip. It's usually much more expensive to have breakfast in the hotel than if you find a nearby coffee shop or deli; for the $5 you pay for the standard hotel continental breakfast (juice and a muffin), you can get enough to hold you past lunch in a coffee shop.

Many people save money and calories by eating only two meals a day when they travel. The bonus is that you don't overdo and feel like a blob from it!

Fire Exits

Always check where the fire exit is in your hotel or motel. If the halls are filled with smoke, it's hard to read exit signs.

Health

If you are concerned about health conditions in the places you plan to visit, contact your local health department and/or the government tourist offices. You can find out about required immunizations as well as any other precautions you should take. You can get a booklet from the International Health Care Service of New York Hospital–Cornell Medical Center, 525 East 68th Street, Box 210, New York, NY 10021. Send a $3 check and a self-addressed, stamped, #10 large envelope.

Hotels

Match your hotel to your activities. A hotel farther from the center of town will be cheaper, but if you have all your business and pleasure in the center of town, you'll spend what you save on the room on taxi rides.

If you want a quiet room, you don't want one that's on the street side or near the maintenance equipment of the hotel.

Find out about check-out time; you can check out and leave luggage with the bell captain while you make last-minute treks around town before plane time.

Always make reservations! And if your hotel has overbooked (as many do), some states require that the hotel transport you to an equal-value room in another hotel and pay for it, as well as move you back as soon as the reservation you made is ready. Many hotels will "apologize" with extras to keep you as a customer, such as free lodging the next time you're in town.

Insurance

You can purchase traveler's insurance to protect yourself in case of lost luggage, canceled trips, and accidents, but before you do so, check out your homeowner or tenant insurance policy to see if you actually need such extra insurance.

Ironing Board

The easiest way to unwrinkle your clothes is to hang them in the shower away from the stream of hot water, close the bathroom door, and let them steam for several minutes. You can also "iron" some wrinkles out by passing the wrinkled area over a hot light bulb. If your things are really crushed, you can make your own ironing board by tucking a pillowcase in with your travel iron or pull one off the bed. Buy a newspaper at the hotel, tuck it into the pillowcase, and—*voilà!*—you've got an ironing board.

Flat garments, such as slacks or skirts, can be ironed on the floor;

just make a pad from the hotel's towels and press away. And there's a bonus here: getting down on your hands and knees on the floor and/or squatting are good limbering-up exercises after sitting in a car, tour bus, or plane all day. Combine your "knee walk" with armstretching as you reach across the towel pad!

Jewelry

Take only one or two simple pieces that go with everything. Unless you feel as though you can't live without it, it's better to leave your most expensive jewelry at home. Why tempt thieves?

In general, it's best to wear your jewelry instead of packing it. Then you know exactly where it is!

Language

Learn to speak travelese.

A "direct" flight means that there may be some stops, but you won't have to change planes.

At your destination, you'll find that "double-occupancy" rate means the price per person when you share a room with someone. A "double-room" rate means the full price of a hotel or motel room for two people.

"Modified American plan" or "demi-pension" means that your bill includes bed, breakfast (coffee, fruit, eggs-and-toast type), and another meal—lunch or, more likely, dinner. Whether or not you eat, you pay the same amount.

"B and B" means bed and breakfast, a cheaper way to travel, which has long been popular in Europe and Great Britain and is becoming increasingly popular in the United States. Local tourist bureaus usually have B-and-B listings. Sometimes you can stay in college dormitories that are rented out during summer vacation; local tourist bureaus also have this information.

List

Carry along an itemized list of the articles in your suitcases, keeping it in your purse or pocket, so that if your luggage is lost, you can provide the list for the carrier right away without a hassle.

Locks

Lock your luggage for double safety: to keep folks out of your suit-case and to keep your possessions in your suitcase by preventing your suitcase from popping open. The best locks are combination locks—this way, there are no keys to lose. You can use the first three digits of your phone or social security number, or any other number that is easy for you to remember.

Long Trips

When taking a trip by car, pack each day's clothing in dress boxes; then you won't have to lug a big suitcase into a motel every night, just your overnight toilet articles bag.

Long Visits

If you don't like living out of a suitcase when making extended visits by car to homes of friends or relatives, you can buy a light-weight fiberboard chest of drawers and pack your things in it instead of in a suitcase. Just put the chest in the back seat or trunk of your car. Other clothing can be carried in the car on hangers. At journey's end, you're ready to move right in—with no unpacking!

Luggage

If you check your luggage on a plane or train, mark your bags with a bow, sticker, shower decal, strip of colored tape, or anything else that will help you identify it fast when it comes spinning along on the conveyer belt.

Always tape some sort of identification onto the *inside* of your bag in case your luggage tags get torn off.

Prevent lost luggage by making sure your luggage is properly identified and ticketed for your destination when you check in at the ticket desk.

Never put anything in your suitcase that you may need en route. Put medicine, money, traveler's checks, house keys, makeup, tooth-paste, even a change of underwear in a light carry-on bag that will fit under the seat.

Of course, you can travel like I do, and not check anything.

Some people believe that two small suitcases are easier to manage and carry than one huge one; also, if one of your bags decides to take a side trip, you'll still have some clothing in the other to wear. Don't put all of your clothing in one suitcase. Distribute it, pack some of your dressy clothing and some of your casual clothing in each checked bag so that you won't end up with a lopsided wardrobe if one of your bags is lost.

Other people don't like to deal with more than one bag. It's really easier to carry on like I do.

When buying luggage, look for sturdy zippers; they're the first to break. Nylon is the strongest material and expanded vinyl is the weakest; the best soft-sided luggage is as thick as tent fabric. Darker colors don't pick up and show the scars of black, graphite-lubricated, airport luggage conveyor belts.

Money

Before leaving on your trip, gather up change and put it in a small purse so you'll have it handy for telephones, pay toilets, and soft-drink machines. Always keep a supply of dollar bills handy, too, for tipping, unless you can carry all your luggage yourself after following my packing advice.

When traveling to foreign countries, check with your travel agent or local bank for money-exchange rates. You may save yourself some hassle by buying at least some of your foreign money in your bank before you leave, where they speak the language you understand. You might not be saving on the exchange rate, but you'll save on trauma if you arrive in the foreign country when the banks are closed or the airport's money-changing facility is crowded.

Also, remember that you can only exchange paper currency when you leave a foreign country, so don't accumulate coins. Exchange your dollars for foreign currency in a bank where the exchange rate is better than it's likely to be in hotels, restaurants, or retail shops. Often, you'll get a better rate for traveler's checks than for cash dollars. Check first!

If you use credit cards in foreign countries, don't expect the foreign exchange rate that's effective the day you spend your money to be the same as what you'll be billed by the credit card company when you get home. Rates may change between the time of purchase and billing.

Ask your travel agent or hotel clerk for a money rate card (not always available, especially when rates are fluctuating rapidly), or figure out foreign money values to the dollar in $1, $5, and $10 increments, then memorize and/or write them down in your notebook for quick reference. If you plan to do a lot of shopping, a small pocket calculator is a must. And don't insult people in your host country by asking, "How much is that in real money?" Their money *is* real money, even if you feel unreal computing its relationship to American dollars.

Most seasoned travelers prefer to prepay whatever they can; this way you don't have to carry as much money, and if you've been saving for the trip, you'll know what you have left over to spend on frills.

Plastic Bags

Plastic bags are great organizers. Here are just a few of the things you can bag in plastic.

Instead of pill bottles, you can pack the number of pills you'll use during the duration of your trip in small plastic bags. You can also use old 35-mm. film containers for pills.

To avoid having to pull everything out of your suitcase to get at something on the bottom, bag all shirts, pants, shoes, toilet articles, and underwear separately. Then, even if you do have to rummage around, all you need to move is a bunch of bags. And your suitcase won't look as if somebody stirred everything up with a big stick!

If you put all the little things you carry in your purse in separate plastic bags, you can just lift the bags out instead of digging around when you go through airport security or customs inspections.

Plastic cleaner's bags can substitute for garment bags if you need to protect your suits and dresses when traveling in the car. If you can't find any, cover the clothing with your raincoat.

For car travel, put a few ice cubes in a tightly sealed plastic bag. Poke a hole in the bag to get a drink of water without fuss.

When traveling with small children, you can put each day's set of clothing—shirt, pants, socks, underwear—in a separate plastic bag, which will also serve as the laundry bag for the previous day's clothing.

Pantyhose protected in small plastic sandwich bags can be used to pad or stuff the toes of shoes, sleeves, necklines, or shoulders of blouses or dresses. I like to put colored pantyhose with the shoes or garment they match so that they're easy to find when I need them. The pleasant plus is that plastic bags protect hose from snags.

Rolling clothes or packing them with plastic bags helps to prevent wrinkles. Of course, you still need to put heavier things on the bottom—and, remember, the bottom of a suitcase means the bottom when the suitcase is upright (when it's being carried).

I have found that dresses or suits left in their dry-cleaner's bags don't seem to crush as much when they're carried in a hang-up garment bag. The cleaners bags seem to keep skirts flatter and cushion the garments when the hanging bag is folded, twisted, and otherwise mangled in the plane's cramped storage areas.

Zipper-closed luggage tends to leak around the zipper area if the luggage gets wet. Packing clothing in plastic bags or placing an old cleaner's bag under the zipper will protect clothing. Once, the lining of my suitcase got wet, and when I opened it, I wasn't exactly thrilled to find red lines all over my blouses and underwear.

Postcards

Type or write friends' addresses on adhesive-backed address label sheets before you leave on your trip. Then, when it's time to mail off a "having a wonderful time wish you were here" card, all you have to do is peel off a label, stick it on the card, stamp, and mail. Even easier than typing out your friends' addresses is to ask them for a few of their personal address labels to stick on postcards that you'll mail to them. And don't forget to tuck some stamps in with the labels.

Premoistened Towelettes

For traveling, premoistened towelettes are a *must*. They aren't just for cleaning up babies and children. They can remove makeup, wash hands, cool you off in hot climates as face, neck, and arm dabbers, or just revive tired, touristy feet. I've used them right over my pantyhose!

Make your own towelettes by moistening cotton pads with a mixture of half rubbing alcohol and half water. Keep them in a small jar or plastic pill bottle. Or just carry a wet paper towel in a plastic pill bottle or sandwich bag for quick cleanup. Tougher facial tissues —the kind that wad instead of dissolve in the laundry—can substitute for paper towels, which you don't usually find in hotel rooms.

Raincoats and Robes

You don't have to waste your luggage space with a bulky robe; you can substitute your raincoat for a robe. A cotton knit or lightweight terry cloth nightgown can substitute for a beach cover-up. Other cover-ups are large baggy shirts or T-shirt dresses.

Repairs

Keep a handful of safety pins of various sizes and a few threaded needles in your suitcase and you'll be prepared if a button pops off or a hem comes undone. A fallen hem can be quickly repaired with tape if you don't have the resources or time to fix it with a needle and thread. It is possible to discreetly hem your skirt on a plane or bus—believe me, I've done it. Also, it saves time, since you're just sitting there anyhow, and you'll look right when you arrive.

And don't forget how handy clear nail polish is to stop runs in pantyhose.

Roll It!

Roll belts, ties, slips, pantyhose, and other garments for neater packing. Jeans and sweaters can be rolled to avoid creases. Some men like to roll one pair of shorts, an undershirt, and a pair of socks together for a daily "packet" of clothing. If the tip of a sock is peeking out of the roll, a traveling man can easily choose the color of socks he'll need for the day.

Shower Cap Substitutes

Forget your shower cap? If the hotel doesn't provide one, make a French twist with your hair and hold it up with your toothbrush or the hotel's pen or pencil (if there is one). Or wrap your hair in a towel, a tank top, a clean pair of panties, or pantyhose.

Snapshots

Taking snapshots of the local children when you travel is fun. You'll get better "posers" if you take along some balloons, chewing gum, or candy to use for kiddie treats. In certain underdeveloped countries and some of the Caribbean islands, it's customary to tip locals who are willing to pose for pictures; check with your tour guide first to find out the models' going rate.

Spots

On most washable materials (not silk), take a damp washcloth or paper towel and gently blot and rub on the spot. If plain water won't work, rub in a little hand soap or shampoo.

You can usually spot-clean a garment while you have it on. The quick trick to drying is to grab your hair dryer and set it on cool or low, then dry the spot pronto. If you are in a public rest room that has a hand dryer, try to position yourself so that it will dry your spot—without turning yourself into a contortionist!

Toothbrush

For a drier toothbrush, slip it inside a clean plastic hair roller or a small plastic pill bottle in which you've cut an opening at the top; then tuck it into a plastic sandwich bag.

You can also blow-dry your toothbrush with your hair dryer so that you don't have to pack it wet and have it taste musty at your next stop.

Tours

Not all tours are twenty-one countries in twenty-one days torture trips. Look for specialty tours, such as those sponsored by bird-watching, gourmet-cooking, and wine groups. For information, mail $3 (to cover postage and handling) to Specialty Travel Index, 9 Mono Avenue, Suite 4, Fairfax, CA 94930.

Unpacking

You don't have to unless you want to! If you are only staying in your hotel or motel a night or two, you may want to just pull out what you'll need, then put it back when you have finished using it so that you don't have possessions strewn around the room and have to waste time gathering it all up again when it's time to leave. As I've said, I like to put things out because it makes me feel more at home. Whatever works for you is the best system to use.

• TRAVEL TROUBLE •

Although Murphy's law (whatever can go wrong will) doesn't *always* apply, it's a good idea to be prepared. There are some precautions that are just plain sensible.

Crime Prevention

Don't ask for trouble! *Do* use common sense.

Do use traveler's checks and credit cards for major purchases so that you don't flash large amounts of cash in public. Keep records of your traveler's checks and credit card numbers in case they are lost or stolen. If you are traveling by car, keep your car registration and a description of your car's identifying marks (dents, et al.) with you at all times. Keep the information in your wallet. Leave large amounts of cash in the hotel safe, *not* in your room. Some hotels even provide safes in certain individual rooms.

Don't keep cash, credit cards, traveler's checks, and keys all in one pocket. If you are traveling with your spouse or family, share the wealth so that if one of you is the target for a pickpocket, there will still be money left to bail you all out.

Do guard your purse if you are a woman. *Don't* put it on the restaurant floor or hang it by its strap on a chair. Keep it on your lap or put your foot through the strap.

Don't hang handbags on stall hooks in rest rooms or put them on the rest room floor; both are easy targets for a quick hand. Place your handbag between your feet with one foot through the strap. Some handbags will fit nicely on the tissue holders and others can be tucked under your chin.

Do leave expensive jewelry and furs at home. If you just can't be without it, you can cover up a noticeably expensive ring, such as a large diamond, by turning the diamond toward your palm. Tuck expensive necklaces inside clothing.

Do keep your eye on luggage in hotel lobbies, airports, anywhere where it can be spirited off by a fast-moving thief.

Don't put all luggage, purses, cameras, or gifts in the trunk of your car.

Do always use the dead-bolt lock and chain on your hotel room door, even during the day. If possible, ask the maid to clean your room while you eat breakfast, and then put the DO NOT DISTURB sign on the door when you leave for the day. When you go out for the evening, turn on a light and leave the TV or radio playing softly.

Don't turn in your key each time you leave the hotel. Keep your key with you; a key visible in the message box—in full view in some hotels—is an indication that you aren't in your room.

Do walk in lighted areas at night; if you think someone is following you with a car, turn around and walk in the opposite direction.

If they turn too, get help. Scream, "Fire." Personal defense experts say it gets more attention than screaming, "Help." Always carry your key or keys in your pocket or hand. If you have to defend yourself, you can use the key as a weapon. The nose (nostrils are most vulnerable) and eyes are good targets for a temporary defense. A swift knee or foot (if it won't put you off balance) to the abdomen or groin area is a temporary defense, just as your mom probably told you.

Overseas Trouble

If you get into trouble when traveling overseas, contact the American consulate or embassy. Their staffs can provide lists of English-speaking lawyers, doctors, or vets (but cannot recommend specific doctors); arrange for relatives to send you money or for you to get a repatriation loan so you can travel directly back to the United States; get you a passport replacement; protect your rights in a court or jail (real trouble!); help you find missing family members; provide notary service; and assist you with absentee voting ballots. It's a good idea to carry along extra passport photos just in case you have to apply for another passport; it saves time and confusion.

If you lose your money or get robbed, a U.S. consulate or embassy cannot give you money to continue your trip. Nor can it cash your personal checks, make hotel reservations, or provide mail service.

Woman Alone

A woman traveling alone in foreign countries should be aware that, in some places, her being out alone at night is interpreted as a request for companionship. The word to the wise is: beware!

If you are dining alone in this country, it's sometimes better to make a reservation so that you don't get caught in a crunch of larger parties getting the tables first. Some dining rooms are not considerate of women alone when the dining room is busy. Make a reservation, plan ahead, and stand your ground!

Many larger hotels have a captain's or maitre d's table for people traveling alone. You can request that you be seated at that table. It does not mean you are looking for company, just dinner conversation.

A dear friend of mine, Donna Mullinex, who has been a traveling newspaper woman for a long time, well before many women traveled alone, gave me some of the best travel advice ever. If you want to have a cocktail or just be around people rather than hibernate in your room all of the time, here is what you might do. When you go into the lounge or lobby bar, tell the bartender or waitress that you are a guest in the hotel, that you are there for a drink, and that you don't want to be bothered or have anyone "send the lady a drink."

In a hotel dining room, I always have a paper to read or make notes in my pad so it doesn't look like I am looking for companionship.

Also, don't be ashamed or afraid to ask a bell or security person to walk you to your room if you feel uncomfortable, especially late at night. They will be more than happy to oblige.

Don't open the door unless you know who is outside. Did you order room service? Can you look through the peephole to see who it is? Once a "maintenance man" knocked on my door. I hadn't called anyone and he wasn't wearing a uniform. When I called the front desk, they told me they had not sent him. He was gone when I went back to the door and security didn't know who he was.

This is why it's a very good idea to keep a chain or lock on at all times; you never know who has a pass key, or who might have one from a previous stay. At night, I even put a chair or place a trash can in front of the door as a home-style burglar alarm. I don't think I'm being silly! I'm just playing it safe.

Women who don't like traveling alone can find singles groups through travel agents or local travel clubs. Get some references about the clubs and attend some of the meetings to be sure you'll be traveling with your kind of people.

Sickness and Health

In developing foreign countries, don't drink the water. Watch out also for hidden water in raw salads, vegetables, fruit, ice, tap water when brushing your teeth. Have wine, beer, and soft drink bottles opened at the table to prevent their being watered down with the very water you are trying to avoid. Often, bottled water bottles are refilled; be sure the one served you has an unbroken seal. Ordering carbonated water is usually a safe way to get a fresh, uncontaminated bottle.

Don't drink unpasteurized milk, and avoid any food that has been sitting out, especially custards, creams, cold mixtures. Avoid those rare steaks you eat back home. Eat only thoroughly cooked food.

Normally water and food in northwestern Europe and the British Isles is safe because of high hygiene standards. Tropical, subtropical, and developing countries don't always have as high standards.

Should you get Montezuma's revenge, Delhi belly, pharoah's curse (or Gyppie tummy in Egypt), the most common aids are Pepto Bismol, Kaopectate, Lomotol, and any prescription you were smart enough to get from your doctor before you left home.

A friend of mine paid $8 per single pill of Lomotol to a Middle Eastern hotel staff doctor, who pocketed the money—four pills for $32. It was a necessary travel expense, but, she said, it rankled her soul. The moral of the story is see your own doctor for aids before you leave. Some antibiotics can be prescribed to prevent diarrhea from ever spoiling your trip. Should your doctor prescribe preventive medication—antidiarrheal or antimalarial—be sure to follow directions exactly, noting if you need to start medicating before you start your trip and/or continue for some time after your return.

The United States does not require immunizations for reentry anymore, but some countries still require some immunizations before you can cross their borders. You can get an International Certificate of Vaccination from passport offices, travel agents, airlines, and doctors. If you have allergies that prevent you from getting certain immunizations, get a signed statement from your doctor that says so.

Your travel agent is a good source for health and weather information about the place you will travel to. Ask and you'll receive the information you need.

A FINAL WORD

Beauty is a much bigger word than I thought it was, because it embraces so many things. It's much more than the way you look. It's the way you think and feel. It involves just about every facet of your life—and that explains why this book turned out to be longer than I anticipated.

You may be overwhelmed by all the dos and don'ts. But I hope you're not; every tip is not for every reader. Be selective and use the hints that help you because, for example, they suit your skin, hair, or exercise needs, or because they fit in neatly with your life-style.

Beauty is all-important because the way you look influences the way you feel, and conversely, the way you feel influences the way you look. Look your best and self-confidence soars. When you get beauty know-how down to a routine—and that's what this book helps you do—you'll find it works right in and doesn't take a great deal of extra time at all. It's easy, and what's easy is Heloisian. I believe in getting things done—but without slaving over them.

BIBLIOGRAPHY

Arpel, Adrien. *How to Look Ten Years Younger*. New York: Warner Books/ Rawson, Wade. 1980.

Audette, Vicki. *Dress Better For Less*. Deephaven, Minn.: Meadowbrook Press, 1981.

Brinkley, Christie. *Christie Brinkley's Outdoor Beauty & Fitness Book*. New York: Simon and Schuster, 1983.

Brown, Helen Gurley. *Having It All*. New York: Simon and Schuster, 1982.

Calabrese, Edward J., and Michael W. Dorsey. *Healthy Living In An Unhealthy World*. New York: Simon & Schuster, 1984.

Cho, Dr. Emily, and Hermine Lueders. *Looking, Working, Living Terrific 24 Hours a Day*. New York: G. P. Putnam's Sons, 1982.

Chobanian, Aram V., M.D., and Lorraine Loviglio, with Patrick O'Reilly. *Boston University Medical Center's Heart Risk Book*. New York: Bantam, 1982.

Dolit, Alan. *You Can Lose Weight*. New York: Nellen, 1980.

Eber, Jose. *Shake Your Head, Darling*. New York: Warner Books, 1982.

Evans, Linda. *Linda Evans Beauty & Exercise Book*. New York: Simon & Schuster, 1983.

Fatt, Amelia. *Conservative Chic*. New York: Times Books, 1983.

Feldon, Leah. *WomanStyle*. New York: Clarkson N. Potter, 1979.

Fulton, James E. Jr., M.D., Ph.D., and Elizabeth Black. *Dr. Fulton's Step-by-step Program For Clearing Acne*. New York: Harper & Row, 1983.

Gieseking, Hal. *The Complete Handbook For Travelers*. New York: Pocket Books, Simon & Schuster, 1979.

Haberman, Fredric, M.D., and Denise Fortino. *Your Skin: A Dermatologist's Guide to a Lifetime of Beauty and Health*. New York: Berkley Books, 1983.

Heloise. *Hints From Heloise*. New York: Arbor House, 1980.

Heloise, *Help From Heloise*. New York: Arbor House, 1982.

Hill, Devra Z., Ph.D. *Rejuvenate*. Hollywood, Cal.: Irwin Zucker & Daughters, 1982.

Hittleman, Richard. *Richard Hittleman's 30 Day Yoga Meditation Plan*. New York: Bantam, 1978.

Instant Exercises. New York: Dell, 1981.

Pinckney, Cathey, and Edward R. Pinckney, M.D. *Do-It-Yourself Medical Testing: More Than 100 Tests You Can Do At Home*. New York: Facts on File, 1983.

Principal, Victoria. *The Body Principal*. New York: Simon and Schuster, 1983.

Scavullo, Francesco, with Sean Byrnes. *Scavullo Women*. New York: Harper & Row, 1982.

Shelmire, Bedford Jr., M.D. *The Doctor's Overnight Beauty Program*. New York: St. Martin's Press, 1981.

Stasi, Linda. *Simply Beautiful*. New York: St. Martin's/Marek, 1983.

Tiegs, Cheryl. *The Way to Natural Beauty*. New York: Fireside Books, Simon & Schuster, 1980.

Wallach, Janet. *Working Wardrobe*. New York: Warner Books, 1981.

Whelan, Elizabeth M., and Fredrick J. Stare. *The 100% Natural Purely*

Organic, Cholesterol-Free, Megavitamin, Low-Carbohydrate Nutrition Hoax. New York: Atheneum, 1983.

Winston, Stephanie. *Getting Organized.* New York: Warner Books Edition, with W. W. Norton, 1978.